BUSHCRAFT

How to Heal Oneself in the Wilderness

BRANDA NURT

© **Copyright 2020 - All rights reserved.**

The content contained within this book may not be reproduced, duplicated or transmitted without direct written permission from the author or the publisher.

Under no circumstances will any blame or legal responsibility be held against the publisher, or author, for any damages, reparation, or monetary loss due to the information contained within this book, either directly or indirectly.

Legal Notice:

This book is copyright protected. It is only for personal use. You cannot amend, distribute, sell, use, quote or paraphrase any part, or the content within this book, without the consent of the author or publisher.

Disclaimer Notice:

Please note the information contained within this document is for educational and entertainment purposes only. All effort has been executed to present accurate, up to date, reliable, complete information. No warranties of any kind are declared or implied. Readers acknowledge that the author is not engaging in the rendering of legal, financial, medical or professional advice. The content within this book has been derived from various sources. Please consult a licensed professional before attempting any techniques outlined in this book.

By reading this document, the reader agrees that under no circumstances is the author responsible for any losses, direct or indirect, that are incurred as a result of the use of information contained within this document, including, but not limited to, errors, omissions, or inaccuracies.

This book is not meant to be used, nor should it be used, to diagnose or treat any medical condition. For diagnosis or treatment of any medical problem, consult your own physician. The publisher and author are not responsible for any specific health or allergy needs that may require medical supervision and are not liable for any damages or negative consequences from any treatment, action, application or preparation, to any person reading or following the information in this book.

If you're in a life-threatening or emergency medical situation, seek medical assistance immediately.

Table of Contents

Introduction 1

Chapter 1: The Wildlife: Insects, Spiders, and Snakes 8

    Insects and Spiders 10

    Snakes and Other Venomous Creatures 28

    Preventative Measures 35

Chapter 2: The Wildlife: The Greenery, Plants, and Other Shrubs 37

    The "Good" Plants 38

    The "Bad" Plants 46

Chapter 3: Wounds and Burns 53

    Self-Healing From Wounds 54

    Self-Healing From Burns 64

Chapter 4: Bone and Muscle Injuries 69

    Fractures 70

    Dislocations and Other Injuries 74

Chapter 5: Food Poisoning and Choking 80

    Food Poisoning 81

    Choking 84

CPR 86

Chapter 6: Emotional and Spiritual Healing in the Wilderness ... 89

Silent Therapy 92

Solitude 94

The Mental Revival 96

Chapter 7: Altitude Sickness 101

Self-Healing from Altitude Sickness 103

Tips on How to Prevent Altitude Sickness 106

Chapter 8: The Backpack 109

Self-Healing Essentials 111

Other Essentials 116

Conclusion 120

Bibliography 122

Introduction

Many individuals are often fascinated by the "outdoors" and the entire concept of exploring the wilderness, however, very few often go out to experience it for themselves. Many factors/things can be blamed for this extremely low participation in wilderness exploration, camping, hiking, and other such activities. The modern, technologically forward lifestyle is one of the factors that is a major obstacle in the quest to explore more areas and lifestyles in one lifetime. The busy office hours in a capitalistic model can be demanding, leaving you no time to devote to your hobbies and other ambitions.

Whatever the reason, now is the time to make an effort towards achieving your goals or exploring your hobbies. The time is right since many people have realized the importance of such activities in the grand scheme of things. Hobbies and activities keep the human mind sane so that it keeps on functioning efficiently when you get back to your jobs and lives. Such activities can also be termed as "escapism" since they allow people to leave their hectic lives for a moment and gain clarity. However, this book has not been designed to discuss the importance of wilderness exploration and outdoor skills. You would not be reading it if you did not think that these skills were important enough to be talked about. In fact, this book talks about using your important survival skills and sharpening them to fight the dangers of the bush better.

These wilderness skills have been given a general term so that it is easier to describe, called "Bushcraft." Bushcraft encompasses the knowledge and skills required to survive in the bush. The world itself is derived from "bush," which is used loosely to describe the forest, shrubs, and other greenery. The craft required to survive the bush was then called Bushcraft by the British and Dutch colonists. The term has also been used in Australia and South Africa for a couple of centuries now. Sometimes Bushcraft can be substituted for other terms such as "survival skills" or "self-reliance" where it seems appropriate; however, the original word seems to be a canopy term that covers the meaning of all other terms.

If you have the opportunity to visit the bush frequently, then you should not hesitate to explore the area. It also presents an excellent opportunity to bond with family and friends in order to form more fulfilling relationships. However, along with the importance of this activity, there are also a few dangers. These dangers can be life-threatening; thus, they prompt this writing. This resource is equipped with the best resources to guide you through your future adventures in the safest way possible. Studying this would also give you the assurance to go the step forward and explore the wilderness on your own.

Bushcraft: Suitability and Accessibility

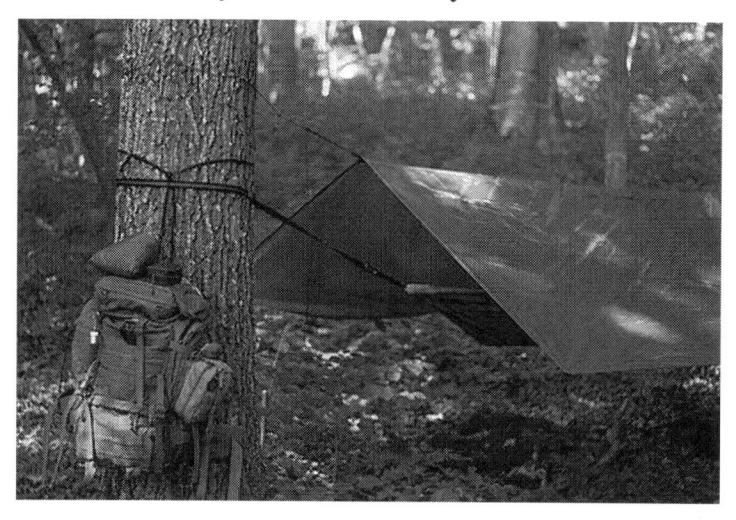

Bushcraft is a broad term encompassing a number of activities, which increases the number of people involved in it. Bushcraft can involve wood-crafting skills, survival skills, wilderness exploration, and even camping! The simplicity is not properly defining the term allows many people to be involved in it without them actually knowing about it. Bushcraft is suitable for anyone that is interested in knowing about the outdoors and has time to dedicate to this hobby.

Essentially bush crafting may be integrated into each of our lives without us knowing. Picking berries, firewood, and other such activities can also be considered bush crafting if you are foraging for survival. Some bushcrafters are strict about following the rules set by wilderness explorers while other amateurs like to dabble at their own will to extract the greatest utility from the activity.

It is difficult to survive in the bush for handicapped people since they may not be able to perform the tasks that an able-bodied human may perform. Performing these tasks is essential to the survival of individuals in the wild, thereby excluding handicapped people from this activity. However, it also depends on the type of disability and the characteristics of the individual. If the disability is not a cause for concern and does not cause huge interferences in the day to day actions of the individuals, then he/she may be suited for bushcraft. It also depends on the keenness of the induvial and if they are willing to overcome the hardships to explore.

Before any drastic decisions are made, an individual should be aware of all the things he/she would be taking on when they decide to explore the bush on their own. The most important aspect of bushcrafting is fire-making. Explorers need to be able to make fires, collect firewood, keep the fire alive, and tend to the fire from time to time. The second most important thing is to forage for food and water. Individuals must be aware of their surroundings and should know what is edible and what is dangerous. Other than these two essential aspects of bushcrafting, the other aspects come from gaining experience in the activity. However, you should decide if bushcrafting is a suitable activity for you based on your willingness to learn the things mentioned above as they are essential to your survival in the wilderness.

The act of exploring the wilderness, however, is not accessible to everyone due to the rapid population growth of the world in the last few centuries. It was a far more useful skill a couple of centuries ago, whereas now, people need to drive for a day or two to access an area that can be labeled as "the wilderness." The need for this lifestyle to exist is immense, as it would ease a lot of personal problems related to mental health by providing a gateway to a calmer world for a few days a month. Many governments have tried to work this problem out and have succeeded in making national parks more accessible to the urban population. Along with such efforts, marking out hiking trails was also seen as an effort to allow more people to participate in exploration and learn bushcraft. According to expert explorers, this activity is necessary to cleanse the mind and soul of worldly obligations and become closer to this Earth. Keeping this philosophy in mind, individuals should make personal efforts to access the wilderness more often to learn about the history of the world and structures that existed long before the building we work in, and the roads we drive on.

Throughout the book, many aspects of bushcraft are explored. The rewarding aspects are far greater than the dangerous aspects of exploring the bush. Due to these rewarding experiences, an individual should indulge in the activity to learn and benefit from it. Accessibility and Suitability are two major factors that need to be ticked in order for individuals to start exploring the wild.

Dangerous Wilderness

People do not need a lot to survive in the wild in terms of tools and other stuff. Some gear is necessary, a knife, a kettle, and of course, this book is all you need to navigate your way through any terrain/bush. It may seem simple; however, it requires a lot of caution as wilderness exploration can be dangerous, and in some cases, even deadly. But this statement should not prompt you to look the other way and run from this challenge; in fact, it should make you feel responsible and in control of your decisions. It should be looked at in a "freeing" manner rather than in a "dangerous" manner because this guide is all you need to protect yourself from the dangerous things in the wild.

Each chapter is designed to deal with a different issue that may arise when an individual is out exploring on their own. The first few chapters look at the wildlife in the bush and how explorers can protect themselves from it. National parks and other bushes have trails marked out to protect explorers from bigger threats like bears and other huge animals; however, encounters with snakes, insects, and smaller threats are much common. It is these threats that are looked upon in the first few chapters and analyzed in great detail.

Other chapters that follow look at some self-inflicted and accidents that may occur in certain areas of exploration. Such accidents may include burns from making fires to wounds from hiking and traveling on foot. Some expert opinions and remedies are expressed under those topics so that your next hike may be a more peaceful one rather than an injury-filled one. Explorers tend to carry a book or two with them in order to solve a bushcraft related issue on the spot by taking things from the wild. This is a similar resource that will allow you to heal yourself from the plethora of issues that may arise on your travels. Keeping that in mind, it will be wise to take keep this book in your backpack before you set out for your exploration.

Another focus of this resource will be on the emotional and spiritual healing that is provided by the serenity found in the wilderness. This is perhaps the most beneficial aspect of wilderness exploration or bushcrafting. A chapter has been dedicated to the explanation of spiritual healing inside the bush. Different exercises and tricks are discussed in this chapter that can help readers gain emotional and spiritual clarity. The source of this clarity is derived from the energy provided by the forest/woods/bush.

The most important thing to take on an exploration trip is a backpack, and the last part of this book covers that part efficiently. The most efficient ways to pack your bag and carry the most important things are listed in that chapter. Some of these items will be important since they will be essential to helping you heal if you pick up a certain injury on your travels. All in all, this is the complete guide to keep yourselves safe and protected on your bushcrafting adventures. It will also be useful when you want to heal yourself from certain injuries and health-related issues (food-poisoning) in the bush. The spiritual healing aspect is also an important read amongst the other chapters as it gives a new perspective on how we look at forests!

Chapter 1

The Wildlife: Insects, Spiders, and Snakes

With all the excitement of getting the chance to explore the wilderness, inexperienced explorers may often easily overlook the natural elements they will eventually find themselves in. Many individuals have set preconceived notions about what the wilderness will be like based on their minimum experience with the wild. However, a major flaw in this norm is the immense diversity that exists in the world, and even in a certain country that makes it difficult for each region's ecosystem to be the same as another. The wildlife of a certain area may be different from where a certain explorer has been before, which is why it is always better to be prepared by researching the next destination.

According to a new estimate by scientists, there are almost 8.7 million types of species in this world (Black, 2011). Some species have gone extinct (from this total number), which has caused a lot of concern for scientists and citizens alike. Due to this reason, scientists, explorers, and governments urge newer explorers not to take up drastic measures that end up destroying the ecosystem while on their camping/hiking/exploration journeys. This Earth is not only owned by humans but by other species alike, which is why we must learn to live with them. This is a major reason behind the importance of this chapter as it teaches readers to treat wounds and bites related to insects and other smaller animals.

Some species have been domesticized but most reside in open environments and natural ecosystems. These natural ecosystems are sometimes part of the wilderness that individuals like to explore; thus, they are taken into consideration in this chapter. Frequent explorers also have the experience of witnessing different species in different regions. This is proof that the number of species stated above is actually true (due to the numerous regions that exist in this world). Most species are indigenous to their regions, creating a lot of ambiguity on how to deal with the threat they pose since different species will have different stingers, venoms, bites, and defense mechanisms.

Other than that, explorers must also learn about prioritizing prevention, as it is always better than cure. Some tips on how to prevent insect and snake bites have also been included to keep explorers safe in the wild. These preventions must be taken seriously since they can help protect explorers against threats that may prove to be more fatal. The saying about prevention being better than cure is very valuable in the case of wilderness exploration.

Insects and Spiders

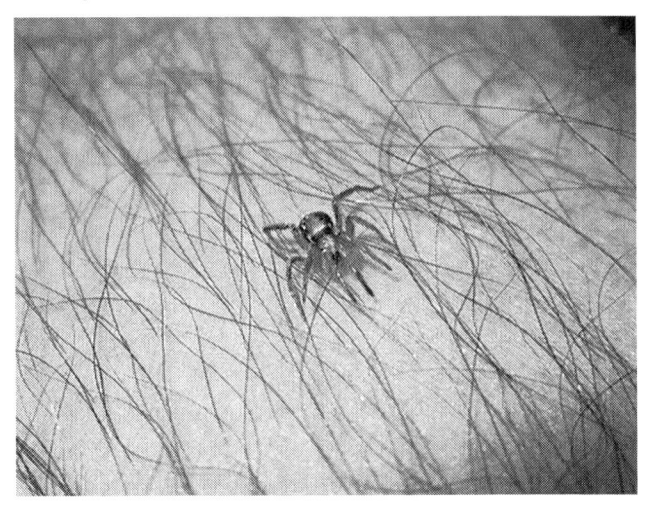

Many green areas that explorers tend to visit will have insects that are indigenous to that certain area, thereby producing a need to find ways to fend off, thus insects and their fronts. The explorers also need to find a way to heal themselves from the bites, stings, and venomous attacks of certain species. These ways are explored in-depth under this section of the chapter on wildlife.

A small first aid kit must be kept at all times if you want to on such an excursion since it is going to come very handily. Not only is it going to be useful in dealing with cuts and bruises (discussed later on) but is also going to be handy in helping explorers heal from vicious bites and venomous encounters with insects. One common class of drugs that are used to treat allergies and some insect bites must be part of this first aid kit that will be carried. This class of drugs is called antihistamines. These antihistamines are common, over the shelf, drugs used to treat allergic Rhinitis. They can be administered in some cases of insect bites to treat the swelling and itching in and around the infected area. These cases relate to different insect bites and are discussed below. The most important first step in all cases is to diagnose the bite/sting in order to find out which insect is the culprit since the treatment varies according to the type of insect.

One of the most common causes of insect encounters in the wild is with ants! Yes, ants are some of the most common types of insects that exist around the globe. The types of ants and their numbers vary from region to region, but there is a well-established way to deal with them. Ants administer some of the sneakiest bites in the wilderness but many explorers ignore them. Some explorers find these bites to be routine as they do not really hurt at all but leave small visible marks that heal over time. Fire ants, however, have a ferocious bite.

The bite left by a fire ant is the most painful one and needs to be treated; otherwise, the journey ahead can be difficult. This bite can be recognized by the small blisters that are visible near the bite area. The excruciating pain that the victim is bound to feel will also give it away. If an explorer feels the pain and recognizes small blisters near a bit mark, it is likely that a fire ant got the best of him/her. The type of landscape an explorer is in can also be used to diagnose the bite. Fire ants are likely to reside in areas that are moist and receive a lot of sunlight. They make their nests amongst the leaf litter, so areas with abundant leaf litter are likely to have fire ants. An example of such areas can be found in the south of the United States. Many excursions that take place usually witness an encounter with fire ants.

It is pretty easy to deal with ant bites and to heal from them. A person can heal quickly, depending on the state of their health. The first thing to do in such a situation is to remove any bits, hair, or stingers left in the place of the wound. These things may come in the way of the treatment that is to follow, which might complicate things later on. Ants bite with their stingers, and the correct process to clean out any stingers is discussed in this section along with bee stingers! The second action that follows is to clean the wound. This has to be done with soap and water, and this step is crucial to the process. Only soap and water need to be used since the typical alcohol swabs will not be effective. In fact, the swabs may be detrimental to the process of healing from an insect wound. Soaps are alkaline in nature, and the human skin is naturally acidic in nature. The soap is going to neutralize the skin and clean the wound more effectively than the other methods of cleaning wounds.

This effectively ensures that the process has been completed; however, there are more measures that an individual can take in order to fight the symptoms that follow and heal from the wound completely. Many victims will face the added effect of the insect/ant bite, which is the swelling. Experts suggest elevating the affected area. This will effectively restrict the blood flow to the affected area, thereby reducing the amount of swelling that occurs. However, another thing must be done before elevating the wound and resting for a bit. Experts suggest applying some pressure to the wound via an ice pack or a cold cloth. This, like the elevating technique, will allow less blood to reach the wound and restrict the amount of swelling.

Antihistamines were talked about briefly at the start, and this is the stage where they may be administered. Antihistamine tablets can be used to help with the itching and the swelling. The body should be allowed to heal itself naturally; however, if you are in a lot of discomforts and the journey has to be continued, then these may be used. Pain relievers can also be administered to relieve the pain if it is too much to handle and is hindering your movement for the rest of the journey. The mention of any lotions and home remedies has been avoided since it is pretty difficult to obtain one in the wilderness. The method has been kept short and easy to follow, given the anti-luxury conditions of the wild.

Any traditional home remedies should be avoided (vinegar solutions) as they are proven to not help with the healing process. The method stated above is perfect for bushcrafters as it utilizes only a few things that are present in all bushcraft kits and first aid kits. The pain and itching can last a few days, but by following this procedure, the healing process will be initiated, and the body must be allowed to heal itself. Doctors do not allow victims to scratch the wound as scratching may effectively risk infection, which will be more painful and difficult to treat on the excursion.

Bees and Wasps

Another common insect that is found on almost any wilderness exploration trip is a bee. Bees and wasps have similar sorts of sting/bite, allowing the healing process to be explained simultaneously. These sorts of insects are found all over the world since bees are the most important insects in sustaining plant life. Bees are necessary for pollination, a process essential for greenery to continue thriving. There are different types of wasps (and Bees) that exist throughout the world, with each region having different names. This reflected in how the Europeans name their wasps. In Europe, the wasps are called German wasps or European wasps. Other regions that are common for bee and wasp encounters are India, China, New Zealand, and the United States of America. Names effectively do not alter the way these insects sting; thus, there is a simple way to act when someone is stung. Bees and Wasps are a common insect that can sting a traveler if their hive is threatened or disturbed. These accidents can happen at any time, prompting the need to be prepared beforehand.

The first thing that is absolutely necessary when dealing with bites from such insects is to remove the stinger that will be left behind. There is a proper way to remove stingers that were mentioned earlier but not explained in detail. The stingers must not be taken out recklessly as the venom may be released into the victim's body. Stingers essentially contain venom that is to be injected into the victim; however, if the immediate responder (or self-healer) is knowledgeable, then this can be avoided. Stingers, if pressed, will release the venom into the body, thereby cannot be removed by fingers or tweezers. The pinching motion of an inexperienced hand or a pair of tweezers can harm the victim. The stinger should be removed by a scraping manner rather than a pinching manner. You can use a sharp knife, a sharp card, or even the tip of a fingernail. The object that the explorer is using must swipe/scrape it against the skin and hit the stinger so that it is taken out from the skin. The first step is tricky, but if correctly done, the procedure of self-healing a bee sting is effectively complete.

The swelling and itching may also be an issue in these types of bites as well. The same procedure should be followed in this case too. A cold towel or a cold compressing mechanism can be used to apply pressure to the wound. The coolness against the skin will relieve the itching and also feel great against the explorer's skin. It is not a great idea to give in to the itching by scratching the wound as it may risk infection. These cooling techniques should be used to fight the urge of scratching. In case there are young adults or children in the group, then a better idea would be to keep nails shortened as this would help in not opening up the wound again if the victim obliges to the itching.

The same idea has been used behind this procedure as well, where easily available things are used to treat the wound to selfheal in the bush. You can carry these things in your backpack or you can find them in the water, like cold water for cleansing.

Individuals who are allergic to bees must also carry a bee sting kit in order to fight off the incoming allergies. The individual should be aware of, beforehand, if he/she is allergic to insect bites. You should always carry a bee-sting kit with you, just in case you or someone else is allergic and doesn't know it.

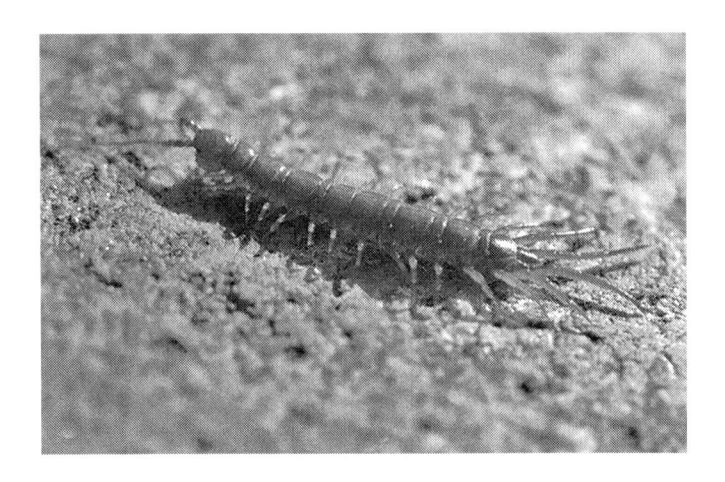

Centipedes and Millipedes

The third most concerning group that needs to be addressed is that of the Centipedes and millipedes. This category is often confused with caterpillars; however, there are huge differences between the two. Other than having lots of pairs of legs and worm-like body shape, there are no similarities. Centipedes are not even insects; in fact, they are Arthropods that feed on plants and shrubs. These small beings are carnivores, unlike caterpillars, who are herbivores. There are stark differences in each of their body formations as well, leading experts to use different techniques to deal with them. Centipedes and millipedes are discussed first, and then caterpillars are discussed separately, within this section.

Millipedes and Centipedes are found on every continent of this world other than Antarctica, of course. Millipedes prefer moist soil and coverage under the leaf litter (usually found in the forest), while centipedes are known to reside in much drier climates. However, both are seen to be found in climates other than the ones described above. Centipedes or millipedes will not necessarily attack travelers and explorers. However, lapses of concentration and inattentiveness by the individual allows them to come in contact with human skin, which is where they can cause problems.

Centipedes are indeed venomous; however, their venom is used for painkillers too! This does not mean that their "bite" will not hurt humans. Smaller centipedes are not of much worry when compared to larger centipedes since they are known to puncture the skin with their "bites." Millipedes, on the other hand, do not inject venom and can be handled safely. Their body, however, may contain poison in small quantities. Sometimes these poisons are harmful; sometimes, they smell like cherries and almonds! Indeed, a certain species of millipedes called the cherry millipede are known to release fumes that are fragrant. The centipede venom and the millipede toxin can be dealt with very easily in the bush if travelers follow the procedures below.

Since these species are not as lethal as some of the insects discussed earlier, the procedures are not as drastic either! Millipedes can be handled safely, and the toxins released are in small amounts. Proper handwashing techniques can get rid of any toxins on your hand or the area that the millipede has come in contact with.

The centipedes, on the other hand, are a bit tricky. The smaller ones, as proclaimed earlier, are not as much of a worry as the bigger ones are. The bigger ones have the ability to inject their venom by piercing the human skin. It is better to avoid them in all cases since it is pretty easy to spot them. If an accident occurs, then the victim may feel swelling and pain for a while. The soap and water washing procedure has to be applied over here, too, in order to neutralize the skin. After the skin has been neutralized, the swelling and pain can be calmed down by cold towel dabs or an ice pack. The pain may not be as vibrant as some of the other bites discussed earlier; however, if it still worries the victim after some time has passed by, then it is wise to administer some painkillers.

The only issue when dealing with these species is to identify which is which. The centipede is likely to crawl away if it senses an external presence, whereas the millipede is likely to rollover. The millipede does not roll away like the centipede; in fact, it maintains its position. This small movement difference can help bushcrafters identify the difference between them. The difference can then help identify which species is safe to touch and which is not.

Caterpillars

Caterpillars like centipedes and millipedes are not such formidable foes. These herbivores usually mind their own business and rarely trouble the explorer. However, as explained earlier, there are many kinds of species of caterpillars, and some of them can be lethal. By lethal, experts mean really deadly! One such kind is a caterpillar from the oak processionary moth. This type of caterpillar might be the scariest foe explained in this section as they travel in groups, arrow-headed by a leader. Their body is filled with grey hair that can cause significant damage at contact. These caterpillars are found in oak forests around springtime.

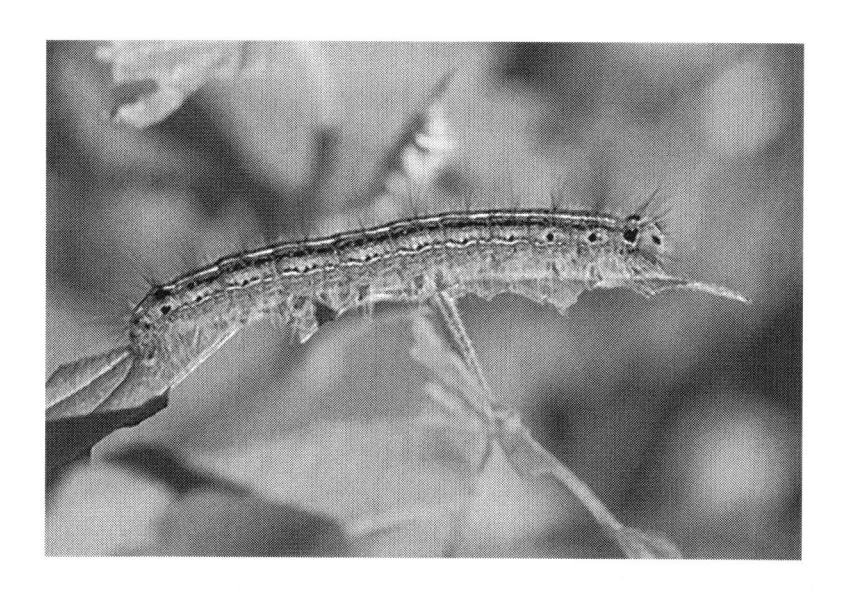

The recommended procedure to deal with such caterpillars is more complex than other procedures. If someone comes into contact with this caterpillar, then it needs to be removed immediately as it may cause more damage with prolonged contact. Experts are very strict about how to remove the caterpillar off of the victim's skin as removing it with hands is a no go since it can cause more damage with more contact. The caterpillar can shed some of its hair at contact, which releases a toxin. This toxin becomes airborne, and as soon as it is inhaled, it can cause conjunctivitis and other respiratory illnesses. The victim may also observe a rash as a result of this event. It is a common sign of epidemic caterpillar dermatitis. The toxin is quick, and the damage is hefty, due to which scientists urge the removal of this caterpillar from the body via tweezers or something mobile, like a pen. They also warn the responders to be diligent and work as calmly as possible, since they could disturb other hairs/bristles on the back of its body.

After finishing this first part of the procedure, the victim should wash the area in contact with the caterpillar with some cold water. It is advised to wash it for a good couple of minutes. It is better to wash the area in contact continuously to rid any trace of the toxin. A good pointer at the event of contact is to try not to inhale until the species is removed from your body. The removal should be done quickly as an average person may not be able to hold their breath for a long time.

Before the cold treatment is administered, the removal of any hair left on the body should take place. The responder can use a sticky tape piece to remove the excess hair. He/she can place the tape over the hair and remove slowly so that the hair comes in contact with the tape. This gentle procedure is the quickest way to remove any hair as effectively as possible. Do not yank the tape or stick it firmly to the victim's skin since this is not a waxing tip! The responder may simply hover the tape over the hair and pull away gently as soon as the hair show signs of sticking to the tape.

The fourth step would be to use an ice pack or use the cold towel treatment to reduce the swelling. This numbing sensation helps in reducing the pain too! Since calamine cannot be administered in the wilderness (unless someone has it), the victim would have to make it work with the cold treatment. Any clothes that were worn during this entire event need to be taken off as well. The toxin may have contaminated the clothing, and they would only be usable after they are washed at a suitably high temperature. This is a safety precaution that may come in handy against the after-effects of the caterpillar toxins.

If the victim feels like an allergic reaction is taking place, that is the effect of the toxin. The respiratory illness would be setting in place and can be dealt with by administering antihistamines that would be present in the first aid kit. Antihistamine lotions are not effective in this case since this is a case where the toxins are inhaled rather than being present on the skin/body of the victim.

Spiders

The next insect on this list is another formidable foe that scares a lot of explorers. Spiders are the creepy crawlers that are feared because of the many fictional tales told about them. The pop culture regarding such creatures has created a widespread fear of spiders that hinders explorers from learning the craft. Learning how to treat spider bites and their venom is a big part of the self-healing process in the wilderness. Many explorers, however, do not know that spiders can be non-threatening companions too! Most of the spiders that are present in the USA are non-poisonous, and you can treat their bites with some of the processes explained above. The procedures explained below will allow readers to tackle spider bites of both poisonous spiders and non-poisonous spiders. The main issue for the explorer will be to identify which is which.

Spiders can be found all over the land in urban areas, as well as in forests and natural ecosystems. They can be found living in trees, plants, shrubs, grass, and any other place they find suitable. Spiders can survive in some of the driest due to their natural evolution throughout the ages. A spider can get its water from food sources, so it is a foe that can be found in most places that are considered prime exploring spots by explorers. However, they do well to blend well with the environment and thus would not disrupt travelers as long as they are not disturbed. Northern America is filled with spiders that are non-poisonous spiders, so it is wise to learn the procedure of treating a bite by a spider. Treating poisonous spider bites is a different procedure and is discussed as well, keeping in mind some of the most commonly found poisonous spiders.

The procedure to treat a spider but that is nonpoisonous is pretty straightforward and similar to the ones that are explained above. The bite needs to be cleaned first, as any other bite would be. This one can be done without the soap. If the victim feels mild pain around the region of the bite, then a pain reliever must be administered. Explorers can also administer antihistamines when an allergic reaction or a respiratory illness starts to bother them. Other than that, these bites are not capable of sustaining long-lasting damage since they are poison-less. Even if some smaller spiders contain poison, it may not be enough to do any lasting damage, and even, in that case, this procedure can be applied. The signs of the poison can be noticed immediately as the pain will become unbearable. The real threat comes from the poisonous spiders, making them crucial to identify from the non-threatening spiders.

In the Americas, several types of spiders need to be avoided by explorers when planning and executing their trips. These spiders are the most dangerous spiders; however, this small number should not be alarming since there are more than 400,000 species of spiders in the world. This statistic makes most spiders less threatening, allowing explorers to be more relaxed. In the Americas, explorers need to avoid the black widow spider, the brown widow spider, red widow spider, and the brown recluse spider.

It is easier to recognize these spiders once explorers know what they look like since they have pretty unique characteristics. The widow spiders have dark-colored bodies respective to their names, followed by distinct geometrical shapes on their abdomen. The brown recluse spider is light brown in color and is very small. It is just bigger than a coin, making it the most lethal small-sized foe in this section. A bite from such a species causes lesions by destroying skin tissues. It is recommended to seek medical attention as quickly as possible if you are bit by one of the spiders mentioned above. However, since there is no medical help in the wilderness, the following procedure can be very handy. Following these procedures may save the life of an explorer or someone from their group!

Black Widow

The black widow is considered to be the most poisonous spider in America and beats the rattlesnake in that category too! However, as discussed earlier, spiders are very small, and their bites may not be very lethal due to the small amount of venom they release with each bite. A healthy person can survive the bite and heal himself from it within two to five days. The person may not even need a doctor; however, it is wise to get the wound checked after the trip is over. It is wise to get a medical checkup after any wilderness trip that is physically demanding. The identification of these spiders has been explained already, and the procedure is explained below.

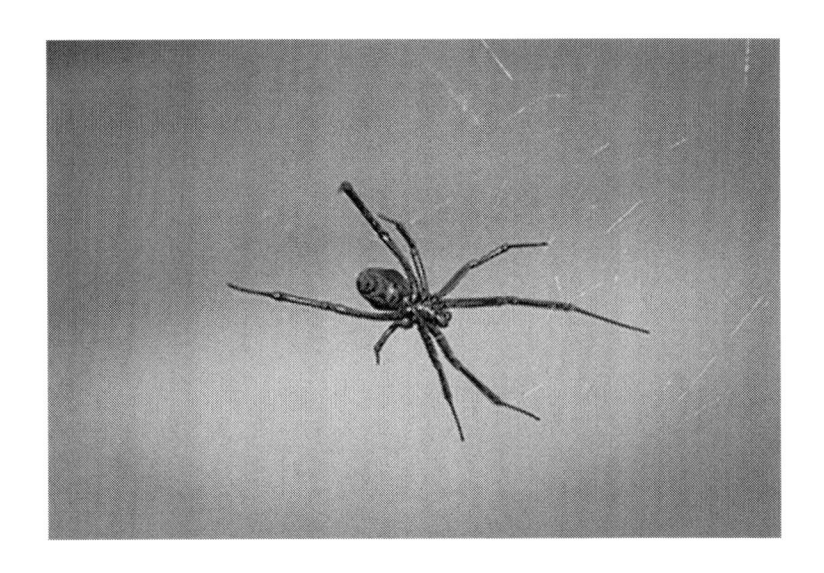

The bite by the black widow is small and painless, which is why it is sometimes ignored. However, the symptoms shortly follow that cause an immense surge of pain through the body via muscle cramps, vomiting, headaches, and hypertension. Any kind of bite should be washed immediately; however, this bite needs to be washed by soap and water in order to make the skin neutral. After this step has been conducted, the limb that is wounded must be elevated. Hold a cool towel or an icepack over it in order to numb the region. The special instruction, in this case, is to lift the limb higher than the heart to restrict the blood flow as much as possible. After these steps are covered, a healthy person may recover soon, but if the pain seems to continue, then some painkillers can be administered.

Brown Recluse

In the case of a brown recluse, the instructions are not as straightforward since the effect of the bite is different. The 0.5-inch long yellowish-brown spider causes a stinging bite that causes a burning feeling, which is hard to miss, unlike the black widow bite. The bite starts as a red spot but turns in to lesions that are filled with fluid as the skin around turns red and patchy. This bite is impossible to miss out on and would need treatment immediately; otherwise, the exploration may come to a halt. In order to heal from a brown recluse bite, the following procedure needs to be implemented immediately.

The basic operation must take place, which involves cleaning the wound area with soap and water. The victim must be immobilized as the activity may cause the wound and the fluid in the legions to cause more damage. If untreated, this dead tissue can expand. The victim must compress the wound by holding a towel/bandage. However, it could be impossible for pain relievers to work this time, and the excursion could be stopped. Immediate medical attention may be required depending on the type of bite and the level of poison administered by the brown recluse. Self-healing, in this case, is possible; however, it is dangerous too.

Ticks

The final insect that is explored in this section is regarding ticks. Ticks are often found in domesticized pets such as dogs; however, they are also very common in the wild. Ticks tend to populate areas of higher elevations in grasslands and woodlands. Ticks are also known to live on and feed on creatures that roam these wild areas. Deer, squirrels, mice, and other rodents are a common host for tick populations.

Tick bites are usually harmless and leave the victim with a small amount of swelling and some redness. However, some ticks transmit bacteria that can cause diseases such as Lyme's disease. This aspect is common in the urban areas, and explorers are less likely to be threatened by tick bites. Having said that, it does not hurt to know how to remove ticks and treat tick bites since some of them may prove to be lethal if they transmit bacteria.

If a tick has bitten an explorer and is still attached to the body, then it must be removed immediately. Victims of tick bites can use tweezers or tick removal tools; however, they have to be careful when handling them. Victims must make sure that the bug is not squished since that may prove to cause more harm than good. Some experts urge victims to remove the tick as quickly as possible to lower the chances of diseases, thereby permitting victims to use hands. The responder/victim must be careful not to apply pressure and crush the tick. The tick must be held from the body and pulled away slowly until the head finally releases from the body. The victim needs to make sure that the head is removed along with the body; otherwise, some more work has to be done. If the head is not removed with the body, then apply an antibiotic cream and bandage the area up.

If the head is successfully removed from the body, then the wound must be treated like any other open wound. The wound must be washed and cleaned up. Antiseptic cream can be applied around the bite if it worries the victim.

The only tricky part in this situation is to make sure that the tick comes off without being crushed by the force of being pulled. The tick has to be pulled apart without being damaged. The tweezers used in this procedure should have fine tips so that they may be able to pull it apart without crushing it. Any other substances, such as a matchstick or alcohol, should not be used to force the tick out if it is not releasing from the body. These substances may essentially damage the body of the victim if he/she is not medically trained.

Mosquitoes and Flies

The last part of this section focuses on protection from the most common flying insects in the world: mosquitoes and flies. These two insects will also be the most commonly encountered species in the wild as well. This is why it is always better to fully cover-up in the wild and carry an insect repellent. There is essentially no hardcore treatment for such bites, and prevention is an effective way to tackle this issue. However, if the mosquito bites are worrying the explorer, then he/she may use some anti-itching cream to relieve the urge of scratching. Covering up, however, is going to help reduce the frequency of bites, thereby reducing the need to self-heal. The body will heal from such bites in a matter of days and sometimes even hours.

The focus of this section is on smaller insects that are common in the wild and potentially dangerous. All types of species could not be discovered due to the enormous number of species that exist in this diverse world. However, most of the dangerous hot spots in the insect encyclopedia were effectively covered, ensuring adequate knowledge on how to deal with wounds. The section also shows what an explorer must and must not do while self-healing in the wilderness conducting his/her bushcraft. If the procedures are followed effectively, then the explorer is well out of harm's way; however, it is recommended to opt for a check-up with a general physician after the excursion has finished in order to be on the safe side since it is a matter of health and life.

Snakes and Other Venomous Creatures

The major threat from insects has already been covered in this chapter, but there still exists a considerable amount of threat in the wild that must be explored. Snakes and other venomous creates, like scorpions, are also found commonly and therefore, must be fought off in order to conduct normal bushcrafting business! The following section explains the dos and don'ts of being a first responder towards snake bites. It is a tricky section that focuses on venom and how to nullify its effect on the body if someone has been bitten. It is an essential aspect of life in the bush and must be read with immense concentration so that all details are communicated effectively.

Scorpions

The first venomous creature in this section is the scorpion. These common desert populations are surprisingly forest dwellers as well. These can be found all over the southern American forests and even in the Himalayas. The scorpions are closely related to spiders and ticks and belong to the Arachnida class of the species classification chart. It is hard to miss out on these creepy crawlers as they have a pretty unique body shape that is easy to spot. These narrow bodies strangers have legs, a pair of claws (like a lobster's claws), and a tail that is used for injecting venom into its victims. The tail is a unique curved vessel that has a stinger on it send that carries the venom. Scorpions are lethal for other animals; however, it is not fatal for humans. Nonetheless, it still hurts a lot, and explorers need to learn how to selfheal in the wild from their stings.

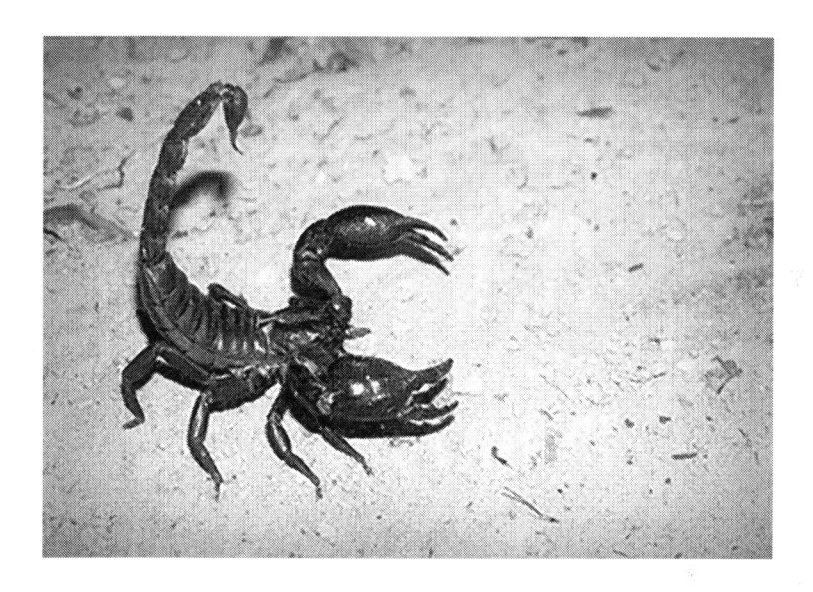

The venom from a scorpion bite can be categorized as a neurotoxic venom. Traditionally there are two types of venoms, neurotoxic and hemotoxic. Neurotoxic bites damage the nerve centers that control essential functions in the human body, such as respiration. Neurotoxic bites can cause nervousness, twitching, over-drooling, and impaired breathing. Without medical attention, the victim might be in severe distress. This is why it is wise to get to the nearest hospital right after the excursion if anyone has encountered such deadly creatures. Even if someone self-heals, it is necessary that experts look at the bite to stop any prolonged damage. The bite, if left untreated for more than 10 hours, can prove to be fatal; therefore, the following procedure should be followed until a trained professional can look at the wound.

The first thing that must be done is to fend off the scorpion with minimum movement. If anyone else is present in the group, then they must do that; however, the victim has to limit his/her activity to ensure that the venom does not spread throughout the body. After the danger of the scorpion is gone, the victim needs to lay down and remain very still. This slows the movement of the venom through the body. If the victim focuses on performing activities, then the heart will pump blood at a higher rate, which is going to spread the poison throughout the body at a faster rate. This is the most important step of the procedure, without which the effects of the poison/venom cannot be delayed or stopped.

The next step is to remove the toxin from the victim's wound. Ideally, another person from the group should attempt to do this; however, if it is not possible, then the victim can turn to self-healing. Experts strongly advise against sucking the poison out as this is the most unintelligent thing to be done in the situation. The sucking motion is going to get the other person infected too! The experts also suggest pouring any substance on to the wound to clean it, such as alcohol. That may cause another reaction to take place that may cause severe damage. The best thing to be done is to use a mechanical suction device. This device can be bought in any medical store, or it may be present in many first aid kits as well. Experts suggest keeping the device over the wound and squeezing the wound area and the suction pump until the poison is out. You can press on the affected area to squeeze the poison out; however, this can only be done until the first thirty minutes, after which the chances of removing the poison mechanically become very low.

After this step comes the cleaning part, any clothing near the wound must be stripped or cut away to clean the wound effectively. The bite area must be cleaned medically, and then bandaged in order to protect the wound from sustaining further damage from the surroundings. This self-healing process is going to sustain the victim's life and can help save it depending on the level of poison in the scorpion sting. The scorpion stinger usually carries a low amount of poison, which proves to be non-fatal; however, it is wise to get it checked from a trained medical practitioner after the excursion is completed. Some snakes have a similar toxin to the scorpions; therefore, some of the procedures discussed for snakes may seem similar.

Snakes

Snakes are the focus of this last discussion in this chapter, the last in this list but perhaps the most threatening and fatal creatures to be encountered on exploration trips. Like spiders, snakes have a lot of different types of species, and it is difficult to account for all of them in a small section. However, one thing that must be noted is that most snake bites are not even poisonous and can be treated on the spot. Having said that, there are a few venomous snakes that can prove to be fatal. However, there is a compact plan of action described below.

Snakes are the most common creatures to be found in the bush and on other exploration trips since some types can live on land and in water. These creatures can survive almost anywhere. Snakes are found in the desert, in the grasslands, swamps, and in forests too! The flexibility of their diet and their bodily capabilities allow them to thrive in most conditions. Some snakes may be difficult to track or notice since they are really good at blending in with the surroundings. Snakes can be found to be carrying either of the two venoms discussed earlier: Hemotoxin and Neurotoxin.

Even in this case, it is wise to end the trip if the explorer knows for certain that the snake is poisonous. There are a few ways to know if a snake is venomous. One simple way is to see how the victim behaves after the bite happens. This can tell responders what type of snake it was, and what kind of toxin it was carrying. However, it is wise to describe the snake to responders as well since that could help in identification and thus alter the treatment plan.

A hemotoxin bite wound appears in the form of fang marks that burn a lot. Some swelling can be observed after the first ten minutes. If the person then experiences numbing and tingling in toes and fingers in the next hour, then it is a clear sign that the snake bite was venomous, and the toxin was hemotoxin. At this point, the common first aid procedure to treat a snake bite will be administered (explained below), and a medical expert and emergency services should be contacted immediately. Some other signs of this bite will be the increase in twitching. After the first hour, if the eyes and facial features of the victim start to twitch is a confirmation that the bite was venomous. Increased heart rate, confusion, tightens are other symptoms. The area of the wound will change its appearance. It will look more bruised, and a person can collapse with such a bite within the next twelve hours. Come common snakes that administer this sort of a bite are rattlesnakes and sand vipers.

A neurotoxin bite can be administered by mambas, cobras, and coral snakes. The symptoms of this bite are very different from what the other toxin does. Initially, only some burning may be experienced and nothing else, which may be misleading. After an hour passes, the numbness and weakness begin. Salivation, twitching and drooling all follow after this initial mark. The victim may feel difficulty in breathing and swallowing in the next five hours. This condition can be worsened by impaired breathing is likely to occur. Without contacting the emergency forces, this bite cannot be dealt with via self-healing, and thus the trip must be stopped. Even though the explorer cannot stop the process, it can be delayed, which may save his/her life.

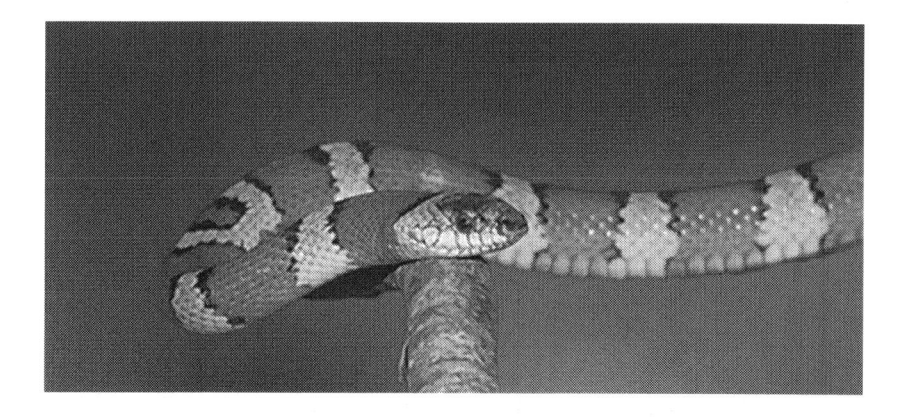

The scorpion bite procedure must be followed in this situation as well. The wound must not be cleaned first! No matter what the poison, the procedure is the same. The identification of the type of toxin is for the explorer to communicate with the emergency responders and other medical experts. The victim has to be moved away from the snake and then kept very still. Without being still, the poison may spread quickly, as discussed previously. The wound must then be the center focus of the responder/explorer. A mechanical suction device must be used to suck all the poison from the wound. Just like the last case, in this case, too, it is not suggested to use alcohol or other liquid to expel the poison from the body. The wound must then be cleaned after the thirty minutes of suction so that any further damage to the wound is not sustained. The rest of the process will be dealt with by the responders that are medical experts. The process for non-poisonous snakes is also similar. The victim can find out if the snake is venomous or not through the symptoms or by visually identifying the snake. If the snake has been identified as poisonous, the emergency services must be contacted; otherwise, the simple procedure must be continued, and the victim is likely to heal from a non-poisonous bite.

The preventative measures are very important in such cases. It is better to prevent a snake bite rather than getting one and then self-healing. Some preventative tips have been communicated below, which will hopefully reduce the chances of explorers being the victims of snake bites and other larger animals.

Preventative Measures

The most effective way to avoid snakes and some other larger animals (like bears) is to follow the trail set up by authorities/previous explorers. Unless you are an expert bush-crafter/hunter or you know your way through a patch of land, it is advisable that you follow the trail set up. Trails allow for more protection for travelers since they have been cleared up. Clearing up the trails from grass patches, weeds, and underbrush removes any hiding places for predators like snakes. This added protection gives travelers less to worry about when they have so much other stuff to look after. Trails are also looked after regularly by authorities/forest rangers, so the surrounding area does usually not host to animals that can hurt travelers. These areas are meant for bush crafters to practice their trade without worrying about larger trails. This does not mean that explorers lose their exploring spirit, if explorers know a place like the back of their hands then it is recommended to explore it at their own will, since they may be experts of their craft.

Another tip for staying protected from the snake, and spider bites, is to wear long boots and hiking pants/costumes. A hiking attire will allow the explorer to move freely while staying protected. Long boots allow the leather to become a barrier between the bite and the wearer's skin. This can be the difference between being hurt or coming away from an encounter unscathed. Experts advise on investing in a hiking attire that will protect you from nature. The hiking attire will be suitable for many climates and destinations as its primary purpose are to cover all of the body to add another layer of protection.

The final tip may sound like the stupidest one; however, it is necessary because some individuals may not know this already. Do not, in any case, disturb a snake. Even if the snake seems dead, do not try to disturb it as it may be waiting for its next prey. The most natural thing you could do is to continue your trip and not to mess with nature's balance, or it could come back to bite you, quite literally!

This section is very comprehensive and rightly so since the situations being discussed are very delicate. It is a case of life and death, so follow these instructions rigidly; otherwise, a negative outcome may hinder future travels. Bushcraft is a trade that is amplified with experience, and this chapter prepares you for the best and the worst kinds of experiences waiting out there. However, the lecture on wildlife is not done yet. There are many other threats present out there than just insects! The chapters that follow talk about other aspects of wildlife, how they can potentially be dangerous, and how explorers can selfheal if hurt!

Note: If you're in a life-threatening or emergency medical situation, seek medical assistance immediately.

Chapter 2

The Wildlife: The Greenery, Plants, and Other Shrubs

Plants are very resourceful for bushcraft. Nature is oftentimes the best mode of survival and also something that can cause great harm to you. For centuries, people have relied on plants for nutrition, and it has made a great component of our everyday diet. People have also used herbal medicine and used its distinguished properties to treat various diseases and injuries, since prehistoric times. However, there are also many plants that are harmful to a human and can cause inconvenience at least, and death at most, to the people who consume or come in contact with it. With both kinds of plants growing alongside each other, it is really important that one knows the distinction between them. With some education about these plants, one can easily identify the different species and tell what is good from the bad. If one achieves this, then their survival expedition can become very easy. This chapter serves this very same purpose and allows you to make yourself familiar with some plants found in the wild.

The "Good" Plants

There are several species of plants in the wild, and foraging through them can be an intimidating task, especially if you are not aware of the different kinds of species. There are a wide variety of plants that are poisonous and should be handled with care. It is important that you do not use your bare hands to handle a plant or put it in your mouth unless you are certain that it is harmless. Even though some plants might be edible, their chemical composition can provoke an allergic reaction in a few minorities of people. Here we will look at some 'good' plants that are safe to eat and useful to treat various injuries.

There is a theory called the doctrine of signature, which was spread from the writing of Jakob Bohme. The theory states that the appearance of the herbs representing different parts of the body are suggestive of the organs they are beneficial for. The theory is supported by the claim that God wanted His men to know what the plants could be useful for. Adventurers, while rummaging for food and medicinal herbs, often abide by this theory. The theory holds true for many herbs, including the stinging nettles. Their hair-like needles characterize stinging nettles, and they are related to stinging conditions like insect bites and allergies. The resemblance of these hair-like needles is drawn to our bodily hair and known to be beneficial for stemming hair loss. Some German brands also used the stinging nettles in their products, like lotions and creams. The products are said to improve circulation and control hair loss.

Stinging Nettles

Stinging nettles are very commonly found in the wilderness of Europe, the United States, Canada, and Asia. The needle-like points of the nettles are located under the leaf and can cause itchiness and redness of the skin. Therefore, they should be handled with care, and usually, a glove or any other protection should be used to pick them. Research has proven that the stinging nettle has various anti-inflammatory and pain-relieving properties. Moreover, the stems of the nettle plant can serve as cordage used for the bandaging of an injury. In the absence of tape, this natural cordage can hold the splint in place, hold the dressing in place, and can be substituted for ropes. The plant is very rich in minerals, like magnesium, potassium, and calcium. It has vitamins A and C and also has almost four times as much iron than spinach. In a survival situation, stinging nettles can be a great nutritious meal. To prepare the nettle to eat simply boil it in salted water and, if available, fry it in a splash of oil. The leaves can also be scorched over the campfire and can consume as-is. The leaves are also used to make nettle tea by boiling them and squeezing the juice out of them. However, in a small minority of people, it can cause allergic reactions, and one should be mindful of this.

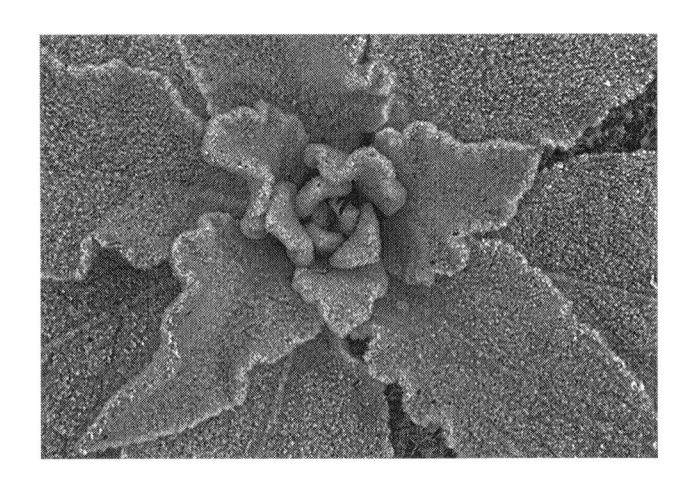

Mullein

Mullein is a plant with huge leaves that are soft to touch and furry. It is a strong plant that bears beautiful yellow flowers. The pale green-grey leaves of the plant and these yellow flowers, which grow around the stem, are a good indicator of identification for this plant. The plant is also good supporting evidence of the doctrine of signatures as the back of the leaf of the mullein plant resembles the lung. The plant is widely known for treating any lung conditions and opening them up in order to improve breathing. The leaves of the mullein plant can be used for asthma and tuberculosis conditions by smoking them. Moreover, the flowers can be used as infusions to treat coughs, sore throats, and tension in the chest. It is also known for treating nausea-like feeling and vomiting. Due to the furry nature of the leaves, it can be substituted for gauze and can be used to absorb any oozing fluids and stop any bleeding. The plant also has some antibacterial properties and therefore, can be used as a dressing. Obviously, it is important that the leaf should be washed and dried before it can be used directly on wounds. Lastly, the size of the leaf enables it to be used as a substitute for toilet paper and sanitary pads. The leaf can hugely impact the quality of experience one will have during their expedition.

Wood Sorrel

Wood sorrel is a plant that can be commonly found throughout the United Kingdom. They have three heart-shaped leaves, similar to a clever. These trifoliate leaves also have white flowers, which can often change their colors to violet or purple. The leaves are no bigger than a fingernail and have a very distinctive taste. The taste is similar to that of an apple peel and a lemon. The leaf is rich in vitamin C and also only meant to be taken in controlled amounts as it contains oxalic acids. An abundance of oxalic acid can lead to kidney complications and therefore, should be avoided. However, due to its rich vitamin C property, it is used for mouth sores and is sometimes used to soothe the stomach.

Cattail

Cattail is another plant that has both medicinal and nutritional value. They are often called a sausage on a stick because of the brown sausage-like flower head at the top. They grow in very damp areas and are found closest to a water source. To harvest the plant, take hold of the base, which is usually underwater, and uproot it. The roots come out along with the stem and leaves of the plant. The white stems and the root, are both edible parts of the cattail plant. The shoots of the plant can be found after stripping off the leaves. The shoots can be fried or sautéed in order to prepare them to be eaten. On the other hand, the plant also has some pain-relieving properties. The jelly-like substance grown between the leaves of the plant can be used as a pain reliever and also serves as an antiseptic to be used on wounds and cuts. It can help slow the bleeding and clean cuts and wounds in the wild. The roots of the cattail can be cut and pounded and used as a poultice for burns and bruises, as well as helping reduce inflammation. The pollen of the plant, the area above the brown cob-like seed, can be cooked to be used as dressing for wounds. It can also help control the bleeding of an injury. Moreover, the brown cod-like seed can also be used as kindling to start a fire because of its dry characteristic.

Burdock

Burdock is a plant that is rich in carbohydrates. It is a very distinctive plant found along with woodland rides and disturbed soil. The root of the burdock is very rich in nutritional value compared to the rest of the plant. It can be identified by its large, coarse, and ovate leaves which have wavy edges. The taproot is brownish-green in color and has a sweet taste, just like its leaves. The root can be boiled in salted water and, if wanted, can be fried to consume as a whole meal. Apart from carbohydrates, the plant contains copper, essential oils, zinc, and vitamins. Historically the burdock plant has been used to remove toxins from the bloodstream. The antioxidant property of the plant also contributes to reducing inflammation. It has also been used to treat various skin conditions like eczema and acne. To treat these skin conditions, the root of the burdock plant should be applied topically to the skin, and the anti-bacterial and anti-inflammatory properties of the plant will work their magic.

Dandelions

Dandelions are highly nutritious plants with thin, toothy leaves about 3 to 12 inches long. They also bear thin yellow flowers, and this appearance gives it its name, which translates to 'lion's tooth.' It is usually found around open lands and fields and grows in rich wet soil. The plant is available throughout the year and is edible from the root to the flowers. Dandelions can be eaten raw or cooked and are rich in vitamins A, E, and K. To cook the plant simply boil it and sauté it if you want. If one does not want to eat it cooked or raw, a tea can be made infused with dandelions. The root is the most nutritious part of this plant and contains beta-carotene, which can assist in combating oxidative stress. The green parts of the dandelion are rich in minerals, including iron and calcium.

Woundwort

Woundwort is a plant that stands out due to its crimson-purple leaves. These purple leaves are easy to spot amongst a wide span of greenery. The plant itself is tall and hairy and often grows along the hedges, wild woods, and the wasteland. The flowers grow out from the central stem of the plant, and the leaves are oval and dark green. The top of the plant resembles a cone, and the stem is longer in comparison to its leaves, which are very small. As the name suggests, woundworts are known for their wound healing properties. It was historically used for this purpose; however, over the years, the popularity of the herb has declined. Nevertheless, it is still a powerful remedy for the injury and helps to stop the bleeding, and its antiseptic properties protect the injured from any bacterial infections. Not only are they used for controlling inflammation, but they are also used for relieving pain. Throughout the middle century, they were used on the battlefield for this purpose. To use the herb for its medicinal properties crush it using a pestle and a mortar. If, in a survival situation, you do not have access to this equipment, put the leaves of the woundwort plant in a handkerchief, and crush it with a rock. Use it topically on the wound to treat wounds and sore. However, they can also be ingested. To ingest the herb for its medicinal properties, crush the leaves using the technique mentioned before and put it in a container of water. Drink the water as normal, and it will help eye inflammation, eye strains, headaches, sore throats, and clear the digestive tract due to its cooling properties.

Curly Dock

Curly dock is another plant found throughout the United States of America. These plants are edible and have various medicinal properties. Their taste is, however, variable from one plant to another. It is most prevalent in areas of moisture and can be found near rivers, marshes, swamps, and lakes. The plant is rich in vitamins A and C, protein and iron. The curly lock leaves have approximately four times as much vitamin A than carrots, which is good for night vision. They can be easily identified by their leaves, which have curly edges, as suggested in their name. In summers, they have red veins and can turn completely into a shade of dark brown. The leaves can be eaten raw or can be cooked. To cook the leaves simply boil them in salted water or scorch them over the campfire. Additionally, the plant is very good for the gallbladder and liver. The plant yellow root can be consumed to increase the production of bile. The production of bile allows the body to detoxicate itself. The blood is cleaned of any harmful toxins. Moreover, the plant also has anti-inflammatory properties and can be used to treat a minor cause of hypothermia and inflammation.

These are only some of the 'good' plants that can help one during a survival expedition. It is impossible to know about and identify every type of plant that you see in the wilderness. However, one can educate themselves and become familiar with most of these plant species. It is important that you read about different species of plants and take the help of someone who is an expert in the field or has a significant amount of experience. If not possible, one should read up on these plants and make themselves familiar with how they look by going through their pictures in either a book or online. After doing so, one should go out in the field and start spotting them and identifying these plants. Feeling, tasting, and smelling them will strengthen your knowledge of these plants and make you more confident in handling them. Learning by doing is the best approach and should be employed before actually putting oneself in a survival situation. Moreover, it is very important that when in a survival situation, one should grab the plant that they are familiar with once they spot it. One should not wait for the injury to occur for them to uproot a plant or go on a hunt to find them. The best medicine is what you have on you at the moment. Making the best use of what you have is the best solution in emergencies. Therefore, do not wait, just act.

The "Bad" Plants

Not all plants are meant to be eaten or have medicinal properties; some can be harmful to the human. There are many plants in the wild that are poisonous and therefore, should be handled with care. Knowing what you are dealing with is, therefore, very crucial. Many people often get various skin reactions when they come in contact with certain plants because they are allergic to them. Wild berries and other fruit looking flowers can sometimes be poisonous and can impact one adversely. We have seen this scenario depicted countless times in movies and books. We will look at some common plants that one should be cautious of and should be handled with care.

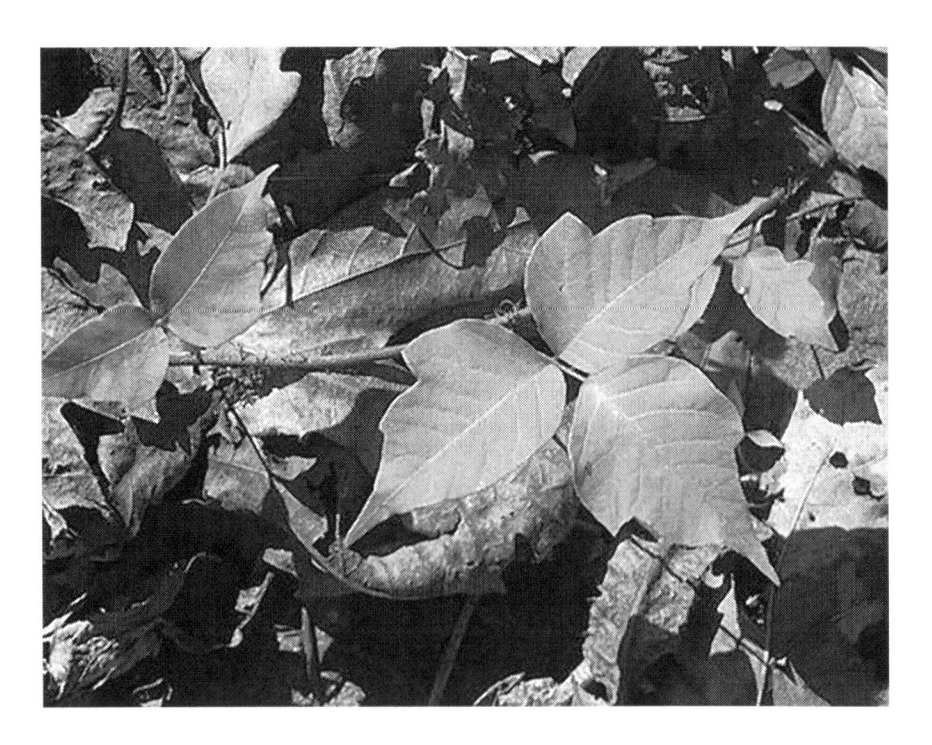

Poison Ivy

Poison ivy is a plant that one will spot everywhere in the woods if they can identify it. The plant is often found in a wooded area and can exist as a shrub or as a vine. The vine can be on the ground or crawling up a tree or any other structure. However, it can easily hide amongst other green plantations and can sometimes be tricky to spot. The leaves exist in triplets and are very broad and shaped like a spoon. The roots, stems, and leaves of this plant contain an oil that can cause contact dermatitis. Coming in contact with this plant can cause an itchy, irritating, and a painful rash on the site of contact. The rash can often look similar to a straight line due to how the plant itself came in contact with the skin. It is important that you immediately wash your hands with soap when you come in contact with poison ivy. If you have come in contact with poison ivy and at night undress and prepare yourself for bed, the oil can transfer to other parts of your body and can transfer the rash. Therefore, it is very important that you constantly wash your hands and pack a sanitizer if possible.

Poison Oak

Poison oak is yet another poisonous plant that can cause an allergic reaction for most if they come in contact with the plant directly. The plant gets its name from the fact that its leaves have a great resemblance to the oak tree leaves. Poison oak is a shrub that can grow as tall as six feet. In areas with shade, the plant can exist and grow like a vine, climbing over trees or any other structure. The plant has leaves that usually exist in triplets but can vary up to nine. The color of these leaves can change depending on what season it is. In summers, the leaves can turn red or green. Moreover, this plant can bear berries of a similar color, which are toxic, like the entirety of the plant. Similar to poison ivy, the poison oak also has oil that can cause contact dermatitis when they come in direct contact with the skin. Research has shown that up 15 to 20 percent of the people are not allergic to this plant and show no symptoms when they come in contact with it. Bumps can appear on the skin of those who are allergic and can later turn into blisters that can ooze liquid. Similar to poison ivy, to treat the reaction in a survival situation, wash the body with lukewarm water and soap. Pay close attention to the fingers and the area under the nails. Also, wash your clothes and change into clean ones after you have washed.

Poison Sumac

Poison sumac is a deciduous shrub and can sometimes exist as a small tree. This plant is very commonly found along with the eastern and southern areas of the United States of America. They are abundant, especially along the Mississippi River. This plant usually grows in wet areas, such as swamps, marshes, and also pinewood forests. The leaves of these plants grow outward, but as the tree grows, the branches bend down. They have an elongated structure and have a velvety texture with smooth edges. The weight of this plant, which can grow as tall as 20 inches, can cause the branch to sag. Just like poison oak, the leaves of the poison sumac plant also change their color as the season changes. This plant also has the same urushiol oil as the plants mentioned prior to this. Contact dermatitis can be extracted if one comes in direct contact with this plant.

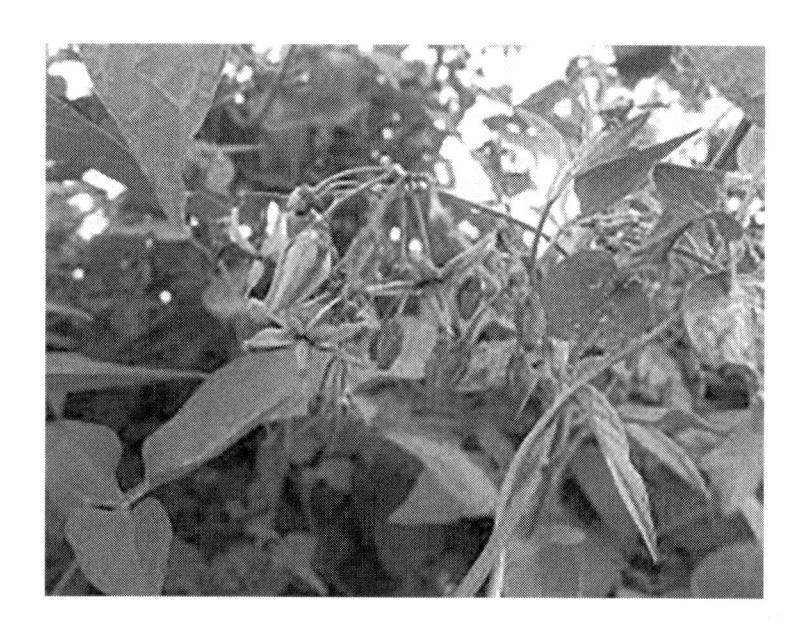

Deadly Nightshade

Deadly nightshade is a very dangerous plant, as suggested by its name. The flower that this plant bears is very poisonous and can cause various complications in a human system. The plant grows a subshrub and can become as tall as seven feet. The plant bears oval-shaped leaves, and the flowers are purple in color. The poisonous berries that grow from this plant are originally green, and they become black when they ripen. Simply coming directly in contact with the plant can cause the skin to irritate and form rashes. However, direct contact is not the immediate threat that one has from this plant; it is the berries that are the biggest cause of death due to the deadly nightshade plant. The plant contains toxins such as atropine and scopolamine. These toxins are capable of causing paralysis and can stop the heart from functioning. Historically the plant was used to make medicine that would reduce the heart rate and allow the person to rest.

Giant Hogweed

Giant hogweed is a herb that was introduced in the United States of America for decorative farming in the early 1900s. It was planted in the gardens and parks as decoration and to add aesthetic. Its large leaves and beautiful white flowers made it the plant of choice. However, it was soon discovered to be invasive and can cause harm to humans. The sap of the giant hogweed plant can cause severe burns on the skin of both animals and humans. The threat posed by this plant also grew because of its ability to grow very big and to spread out over a large area and tangle with other plants. The plant grows to a height of almost 15 to 20 feet and produces clusters of white flowers that assemble like an umbrella. It is usually found near wet soil near farms and swamps. The entire plant is not dangerous; it is only the sap that exists in the leaves and stems of this plant that can cause any harm. When this sap comes in contact with your skin, it starts a reaction called phytophotodermatitis. This damages the DNA and alters the protection mechanism of the skin against ultraviolet rays. The ultraviolet light can then cause severe blisters, scars, and burns to the site of skin exposed to the sap from this plant. The longer the sap sits on the skin, the harsher the burns will be. Moreover, if the sap manages to get in one's eye, it is capable of causing permanent or temporary blindness. The plant can easily be identified by the dark purple-red blotches and the thin, white bristles along the stem. Wash the area of exposure with soap and warm water as soon as you come in contact with the sap of a giant hogweed plant.

Although most of the plants can be classified into two of the categories that we just explored, some plants are more difficult to categorize under these two labels. The holly is one of these many plants that have some 'good' attributes and some 'bad' attributes. These plants can exist as shrubs and can grow into deciduous trees. The holly plant has glossy leaves and bears flowers that are green-white in color. It is an evergreen tree that can grow as tall as fifteen feet. This tree bears beautiful red berries that appear to be very inviting. Birds eat these berries, and this might make you think that a human can also eat the berries of this tree. However, birds and humans can tolerate poison to varying levels, and what might be edible for a bird might not be for a human being. These red berries contain various toxins and can be harmful to a human. Although it is rare that it can kill someone, there have been recorded deaths due to the consumption of these berries. However, one might think that the poisonous nature of this plant could be enough to categorize it under the label of 'bad' plant. However, the plant has certain uses that can ease one's survival expedition. The holly tree has very thin and long branches. The size of these branches makes it good for kindling. It is possible for one to find many of these twigs and collect them at once. Moreover, these woods contain a wax-like substance that burns well. Additionally, the holly tree can provide good shelter for one to camp under. The green canopy of the tree can provide a shaded and waterproof shelter. Some of these trees have canopies that can be closer to or reaching the ground; in such cases, it can provide a discreet shelter if one does not want to draw too much attention. The smoke from the bonfire is also dispersed by the canopy of the holly plant and allows one to stay warm while still being discreet.

Note: If you're in a life-threatening or emergency medical situation, seek medical assistance immediately.

Chapter 3

Wounds and Burns

Skin is a continuous layer of soft and flexible tissues that makes up the largest organ system of the human body. The delicate nature of skin and the fact that it is continuously in direct contact with the surroundings makes it a common site to incur injuries. Any sharp objects, rough contact, high-pressure impacts, etc. can cause the skin to damage. Wounds, bruises, and burns are very common injuries for a human to incur, both indoors and outdoors, especially in an outdoor survival condition, the probability of incurring such injuries increases. The unexpected and unfamiliar nature of the terrain can present various scenarios that can lead to one getting a wound or burning themselves. These injuries can range from a simple cut that is harmless to a gash that can be life-threatening.

Imagine you are planning to camp on an abandoned island in the middle of nowhere for three days. This island is only accessible through a boat, but you do not own one. However, you find someone who owns a boat and is willing to give you a ride to the island in exchange for money but is not willing to rent his boat out to you. You agree to this transaction and schedule to be picked up after 3 days at the same location where he will drop you. There is no cellular reception on the island and no means of contacting the outside world, which means you are solely responsible for yourself during these three days. What happens if you injure yourself on the very first night, and your injury requires immediate attention?

In a survival setting, the possibility to immediately visit a doctor is not present. In fact, in certain cases (like this), it is impossible for the campers to evacuate immediately and seek help. You are your savior. Therefore, it is extremely necessary that one knows how to treat these injuries when they occur. One should also know to pack responsibly and keep things that can come handy to treat any possible injury. The following chapter will explore the treatment of wounds and burns in a survival situation where access to a doctor is not available.

Self-Healing From Wounds

Wounds are one of the most common types of injuries. Cuts, scratches, and scrapes can all leave you with punctured skin, causing you to have wounds. One can get wounds indoors and outdoors, but in a survival setting, incurring a wound becomes even easier. Tripping on a branch, slipping down a slope, or grazing your body against any rough surface can leave you with a wound. Although such injuries might leave you with minor cuts that can heal on their own, they can become dangerous if not treated. Not treating a wound can cause it to become infected and can lead to sepsis, which is a life-threatening condition. However, deep cuts are serious and will not heal themselves. Deep cuts might bleed intensively and need proper care and attention.

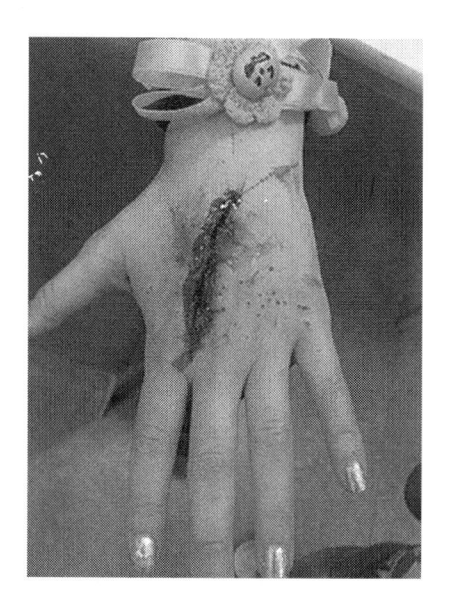

Bleeding

A wound might lead to bleeding if the skin is broken. The first step into creating a wound is to stop the bleeding so that the wound is visible, and the damage can be further examined. It is only after the bleeding has stopped that the wound can be cleaned of any bacteria or dirt. Direct pressure should be applied to the wound to stop the bleeding. Gloves are the preferred material to be used while applying hard pressure to the site of the wound. However, if a glove is not available, a towel, a blanket, or a plastic bag can be used. Bare hands should not be used to stop the bleeding directly unless any non-permeable material is not available. Bare hands should be used as the last option, and only if the injured person is known to the helper and has no diseases that can be transferred through blood. Pressure needs to be applied to the site of the wound for 5 to 10 minutes to stop it from bleeding. If possible, the site of the wound should be raised above the level of the heart. This causes the bleeding to slow down and makes treating the wound easier. If, after 10 minutes of applying elevation and direct pressure to the wound, the bleeding does not stop, apply pressure to the artery between the site of the wound and the heart. Pushing the artery against the bone, while applying direct pressure and elevation, stops the bleeding. These arteries are found on your neck, wrist, groin, behind your knee, near your ankle, your elbow, and at your temples. To check if the bleeding has stopped, slowly release pressure from the artery. If even after following all these steps, the bleeding does not stop, you have to apply a tourniquet. It is a device to apply pressure to large vessels in order to limit the bleeding. It is used as a last choice and, if not done right, can lead to amputation of the injured site. One should not use a rope or a wire to make a tourniquet. A sterile piece of cloth or a large plastic bag should be used. It should be placed 2 inches above the site of the wound and tightened until the bleeding has stopped or visibly slowed down. It shall only be taken off until a professional is available to tend to the wound. Moreover, if the injured person has already lost a lot of blood, it is possible that they might lose consciousness and might start to breathe heavily. In such scenarios, it is important to keep them warm and try to keep them awake.

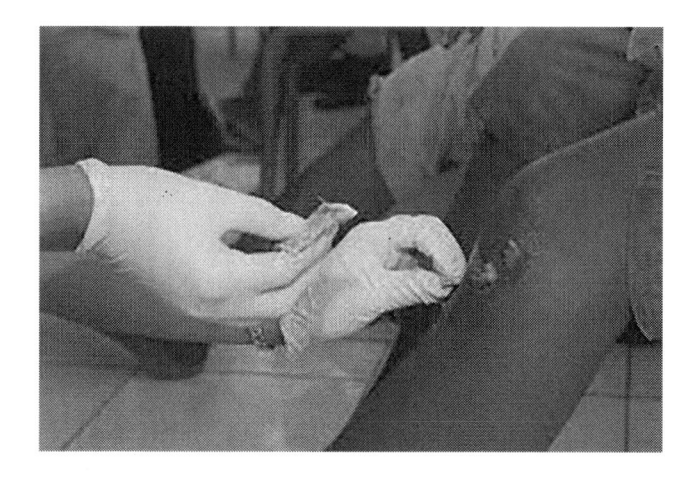

After the bleeding has successfully stopped, the wound needs to be cleaned thoroughly. Remove any dirt or debris from the skin with a clean wet towel. Once you have cleaned the debris from around the wound, pour potable water at a 90-degree angle over the wound. This will remove any dirt and debris that might have gotten inside the wound. It is absolutely important that clean water is used, as water from a lake, pond, or stream could have bacteria that can further aggravate the wound. If you are with someone and injured, have the other person boil the water in order to sterilize it while you attend to your wound. However, sometimes, you may be alone and the best thing to do is find a clean source of water and use it to wash the wound out.

Emergency medical technicians often use syringes to spray water on the wound to clean it. It is advisable that you pack a 20 cc syringe for your adventure. However, if you do not have a syringe on you, you can use a bag and cut a hole in it to act like a syringe. Additionally, one can also use soap to clean around the wound; however, make sure that it does not get in the wound, or it might sting. It is best if the person injured cleans their own wound as they would know best about the pain they are experiencing. The wound might start bleeding again upon cleaning. If it does, then direct pressure needs to be applied until the bleeding stops. After washing the wound with water, apply antiseptic to the wound. Iodine kills bacteria and can prevent the wound from becoming infected; however, in the absence of any antibiotics, one can use pine sap. It is antibacterial and has antiseptic and antibacterial properties. You can collect pine sap from a broken pine branch or collect it directly from the pine bark.

It is important to know that most wounds should be allowed to heal naturally and that they do not need to be closed. Wounds that are incurred in areas of high activity, like the joints, should be healed as any movement is more likely to cause the wound to break open and limit any healing. Other than joints, forehead, butt cheeks and feet are sites where the wound should be closed. Butterfly bandages can be used to close the wound. In case these bandages are not available, one can cut strips of a gorilla or medical tape to hold the open wound together. In case of wounds at not a high movement part of the body, it is not advisable to close it as some microorganisms might still be present even after cleaning. Closing the wound prematurely increases the chances of infection to go unnoticed and makes it difficult to be treated. Even in cases of a serious wound, it is advisable that it should not be closed, and one can get stitches even after a few days. This can allow you to monitor any infections and pus that might form over time, and you can clean it again.

After you have cleaned the wound and closed it, if required, then you need to dress it and apply bandages. The dressing is a sterile pad that is used to compress the wound in order to promote healing. Gauze or a sterile piece of cloth can be used for dressing. If nothing is available, you can boil a piece of cloth and allow it to dry, then fold and use as a dressing. This process must be done as cleanly as possible. It is advised that one washes their hands before and after the process. Once the dressing is applied, it has to be secure with a bandage. A duct tape, gorilla tape, or any material that can do the job can be used in a survival situation. It just has to be clean, and the material has to be tied around the dressing in a manner that circulation is not restricted. Paleness of the skin around a bandaged wound, nails turning blue, and feeling cold are signs of restricted circulation. Limbs below the wound might be difficult to move in these circumstances, and it means that it has to be bandaged again. The dressing should be changed every 12 hours, and it should be done carefully. The dressing can stick to the wound, and it is necessary that it is dealt with cautiously. Not being careful can cause great discomfort to the injured person and might reopen the wound and start bleeding again.

Infection

If there are any signs of pus, infection, or the injured area turning red it means that the wound has to be cleaned and should be left open for a while. If the infection is spreading, the person might get a fever; it is the reaction of the body to combat the infection as certain bacteria cannot survive under high temperatures. In such cases where the infection has been spreading for more than 10 hours, it is capable of causing great damage to the human. One should immediately plan an immediate evacuation and try to tend to the infected wound. Antibacterial cream should be applied, and if not available, pine sap or any other substitute with antibacterial properties should be used to treat the wound. Extracting pus from the wound is also a way to draw out bacteria. Cut open the wound, remove the pus, clean it, and rebandage it every 12 hours. However, it is very difficult to treat a spreading infection in a survival setting without proper aid; therefore, one should prioritize an evacuation plan.

One tends to use sharp objects like knives and axes in the woods. Knives are used for cutting and preparing food, while axes can be used to collect wood for the fire and cut animals hunted for food. Sometimes one can hurt themselves with these objects, and the gash that they cut from an injury with these objects is a clean, open wound. To stop the bleeding of such cuts all the steps mentioned above should be used, however, to be quick, one can use tampons and sanitary pads to stop the bleeding. Super glues are available in the market and have been approved to be used on the skin by several regulatory authorities. The United States' Food and Drug Administration (FDA) has certified many types of glue to be used on the skin. Some brands include Dermabond and SurgiSeal. It is recommended that one of these should be packed and kept in the first aid kit. Minor, clean wounds can be sealed with such glues very effectively. They dry easily, thus stopping the bleeding and successfully keeping air out of the wound. Moreover, it also limits scarring once the wound is healed. This can be used as a substitute for stitches and is less painful than getting stitches. However, super glue should not be used on animal bites, deep punctures, burns, and irregular wounds.

In some cases, the tendons might have been injured, which can compromise the function of the limbs. Tendons are fibrous tissues that connect the muscle to the bone and are composed of collagen. In the case of a deep cut, it is probable that tendons might have been damaged if the limb cannot be moved. The inability to move the thumb after a deep cut to the site probably means an injured tendon. It is to check the movement of the site after the injury is incurred in order to evaluate any damage to the tendon. In case of injury to the arm or the hand, you can use the grip test to evaluate this. The injured person should be able to firmly grip your thumb, even though the grip is not strong due to the injury. Similarly, in case of an injury to the feet or the leg, you can put some weight on the injured person's feet and ask them to lift it. It can be your hand or any other liftable weight. It will allow you to examine the strength the limb has and if the blood circulation is compromised. If, after your examination, you are certain that the tendon is injured, splint the wound, and it should heal on its own.

Blisters

Moreover, blisters are also fairly common types of injuries that can cause discomfort to the adventurer and spoil their experience. It is when a pocket of fluid appears on the top layer of the skin due to friction due to rubbing or even freezing. Most blisters will be filled with plasma, blood, or even pus. One's shoes are the real causes of blisters. When the sole of the boots and socks rub against one's feet, they cause the thicker outer layers to move more than the layers of skin underneath. This causes the skin to break and eventually fill up with fluids. This can more simply be explained by one rubbing the skin of peach with their finger. As the force of one's finger increases, the skin of the peach starts to wrinkle and eventually breaks. Similarly, the outer layer of the skin, epidermis, can break due to friction. The fluid that accumulates is pushed against the skin and therefore causes a bump, which can cause a lot of pain.

To prevent blisters, one should tackle the primary cause that is a poor pair of shoes. It is extremely important that while shopping for hiking boots, one buys a pair that fits them perfectly. In case you choose to buy a pair of boots that are made out of leather, make sure you break them in so that they do not cause any inconvenience on the trip. Wear them a lot before the trip and put it through all the tests you possibly can. One can also use duct tape to provide padding to the areas that are at potential risk of tearing open. The side of the skin and the area above the heel are sites that are common for blisters.

After shoes, one needs to be wise about making decisions about what kind of socks they choose to wear. One should avoid wearing cotton socks at all costs during hiking. Cotton can hold moisture for long periods of time, and if one chooses to wear socks made of cotton, this moisture is held very close to their skin. The foot can slip around in the shoe, and this can accelerate the process of blistering. Wool is the best choice for socks material, as it has the ability to prevent odor and moisture. Even when the socks get wet, wool retains all its insulating properties and prevents blisters. In a survival situation, the terrain is often rugged and unpredictable. There are uphills and downhills, which can be tricky to get past. Going downhill is when your feet move around in the shoe the most. This when most friction between the feet and the shoe is produced, and blisters are formed. One should make sure that their shoes are tightened before they head downhill. If needed, one should pad their feet to reduce any friction.

It is advised that one should carry two pairs of socks. When the first pair gets wet, remove it and change into the other, dry pair. Hang the wet pair of socks from your backpack so that it can dry and can be used later. One should also wash their feet when possible. Long hikes and trails can make your feet sweat and make them dirty. Dirty feet can blister easily, and also it is more probable to get infected and cause greater problems. Therefore, wash your feet or rinse them in running streams of water or lakes. This cleans not only one's feet but also the cold or warm water that can provide great relief to the tense foot muscles. The only one needs to be mindful about is that one should dry their feet thoroughly after they have washed them, before putting their hiking boot back on.

Blisters do not only appear on the feet, but they can also appear on the hands. Blisters appear on the hands because of the same reason, which is friction. Intense repeated motions while handling, tools, wires, ropes, etc. can cause blisters on the hand. To protect the hand from this kind of friction, one should wear gloves when carrying out tasks that involve repeated hand movements. They can also cover that site that is starting to heat up with duct tape. The heating up of a certain part when carrying out repetitive motions is an indication of a blister forming. One should also be on a lookout for any signs of infection once a blister appears. Any kind of redness or red streaks originating from the site of blisters or greenish pus can be indications of an infection.

One might think that popping a blister open is a really bad idea. However, if one continues to walk or use the same repeated motion, these bumps might burst open on their own. It is for this reason that it is advised that these blisters should be split open in controlled scenarios rather than allowing them to rip open on their own. To open a blister and to drain it of any fluid, you need to firstly find a spot to sit down and relax. Clean the blister with soap and apply antiseptic if available, then sterilize a knife, pin, or any other tool you are using to carry out this task. Pierce the blister at the bottom and push the fluid down and out of the skin. Carry these downwards movements until all the fluid and has been fully removed and bump has flattened. Use sterile sources of water to help you flush out any pus or blood from the bump. After you have flushed out the fluid, disinfect the area, dry it and put a dressing on it.

Note that blisters caused due to burns should not be popped. The treatment of burns is further discussed below.

Self-Healing From Burns

Cooking in the woods and putting up a fire at night is a necessity to survive. It is possible that one car incur burns either due to recklessness or a stupid mistake. The degree of harm due to an injury from a burn can vary. It can either be a minor burn from touching a hot cooking pot or a major injury when the sizzling grease pours over you and seeps into your boot. Even a slight burn can cause great discomfort, and they are the worst type of injury you can be subjected to in wilderness. Therefore, it is important that you are prepared to deal with the situation if it occurs since they are harder to handle in the absence of proper medical care.

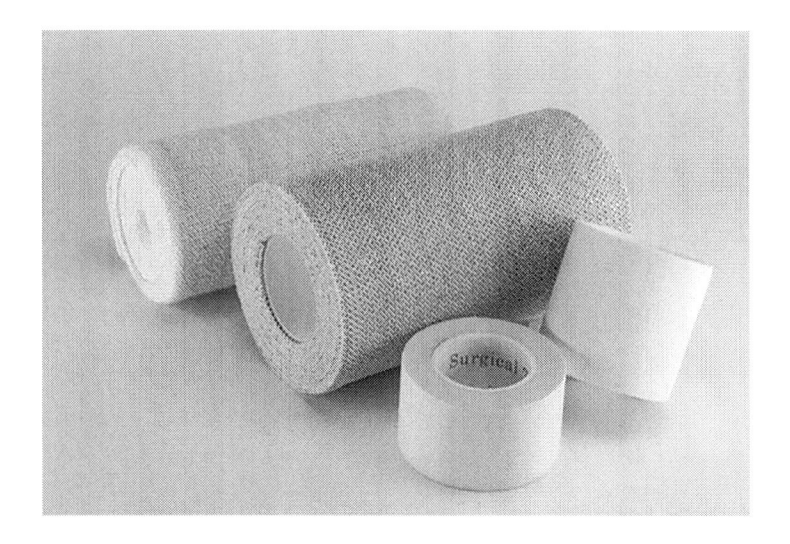

In cases of major burns, like when a person falls into the campfire, your first reaction should be to stop any burning that might still be happening. It is often the clothes that catch fire, and one should roll the person on the ground and try to stop the fire with a towel, sand, or water. If the person is wearing many layers, then it is advised that the additional layers should be taken from the injured person's body. These layers can trap the heat from the burn between the layer and cause further damage to the wound site. However, it is important that the immediate layer of the skin should not be taken off. It should first be examined if the layer of clothing has stuck to the skin or not, in case it has then the wound should be allowed to cool with cold water before any further action. Often when boiling water seeps into the boot, people make the common mistake of taking the shoe and the socks off. Taking off the socks peels off the skin upon removal. The sock and the burn should be allowed to cool first. Water is the best source to cool the burn and gives the injured person great relief. As stated earlier, clean and sterile sources of water should be used. If the burn has not torn the skin, then any cool source of water can be used as it will not penetrate the skin and cause any kind of bacteria to contaminate and infect the burn wound.

Treating Burns

In an emergency situation, when any immediate sources of sterile water is not available, wet and cool soil along with wet leaves can be used. However, they should be placed in a clean plastic bag or an impermeable article. Moreover, if the damage from the wound has affected more than 10 percent of the body, cooling the wound should not be prioritized. Cooling such burns can cause hypothermia because of the unexposed wound site and the absence of the protective skin that provides thermoregulation. Hypothermia can lead to an increased probability of wound infection; therefore, cooling expansive burn wounds should be avoided at all costs despite the relief that cool water can bring to the injured person.

The next step is to clean and cover the wound with a dressing. Use the same procedure as cleaning the wound to clean a burn wound. It is advised that a dry dressing be used only in cases, the burn has penetrated the first layer of the skin or is an uncomfortable location and causing great pain, should you use a moist dressing. In cases where the burns expand over more than 10 percent of the body area, the moist dressing should be avoided at all costs as it increases the chances of hypothermia. One should definitely pack gauze as it can come handy in the treatment of several injuries in the wilderness. You can use the gauze, fold it, and place over the burn wound to dress it. However, to apply a moist dressing, which can cause great relief to the injured, slightly damp the gauze with sterile water and place it over the burn wound. The moist dressing should also be applied to oozing wounds because dry dressing can stick to the wound and can tear the wound open upon removal, thus disrupting the healing process.

In the absence of gauze, one can use a bandana, cut a towel, a handkerchief, or even cut a sanitary pad to use in place of a gauze. It is important that you improvise and think smartly in these situations. Nothing is off-limits as long as they are getting the job done. Deciding whether to apply a dry or a moist dressing to a burn wound can become easier if one is aware of the different classes of burns.

First-degree burns do not break the skin and are comparable to sunburns. The impacted area turns red and stings. To identify it, one can press the center of the burn, and it should turn white, and upon removal of the pressure, it should become red again. Such wounds do not require any dressing and should be cooled with cold water.

Second-degree burns are partial-thicken burns that have melted the first layer of skin. The dry dressing should be applied to these burns unless there is visible oozing of the wound.

Third-degree burns are also partial-thickness burns that have melted all the layers of the skin and are very severe. They require immediate professional care, and until such help is received, the moist dressing should be applied to restrict the pain. In cases where the pain is intense, painkillers should be given to the injured like ibuprofen. *Seek medical help immediately!*

Moreover, when the protective covering is melted, fluid can ooze out from the burn wound, and the body can lose water. In a third-degree burn or when an expansive area of the body has been burnt, one can often face dehydration. The destruction burns can cause to the nerves can affect the mechanism of water loss from the body and thus lead to dehydration and cause an imbalance in the level of electrolytes in the body. Therefore, the injured person must be made to drink water to replace what is being lost from the body. The bigger the burnt area, the more water is lost from the body of the injured person.

When one incurs an injury, it is important that they make the right decisions. To make the right decision, you need to think logically and not act on your impulses or allow the pain you are experiencing to drive your decision-making ability. Therefore, it is very important that you remain calm in such situations and trust your companion if you have any.

Note: If you're in a life-threatening or emergency medical situation, seek medical assistance immediately.

Chapter 4

Bone and Muscle Injuries

Injuries to the bones, including fractures, are some of the most common injuries that take place outdoors. In the wilderness, the terrain is rugged and wilder, it is not designed to be inhabited, and therefore the accidents increase in such settings. Slipping down a trail, falling down heights and falling down trees can lead to injuries to the bone.

There are 206 bones in the human body, and all of them can be broken; however, fractures along the lower arm, upper arm, lower leg, and upper leg are the most common. However, it is just a myth that only harsh impact can cause bone injuries; one can also injure their bones due to repeated activity. This is called stress fracture, and they are either a small crack or a bruise on the bone. They are most common among athletes who run a lot and also among people who are not used to intense activity. Over the years, mankind has developed various treatments to treat bone injuries. Although this injury is painful and requires immediate attention, it is possible to be treated if it happens in the wilderness, and there is no help readily available. The following chapter explores the treatment of various bone injuries, including fractures and possible ways to treat them in the woods.

Fractures

Bones can break anywhere in the body, and they can break at any angle. Fractures are the most serious kind of bone break. It is when the bone has partially been broken, and there is a considerable crack, or it has broken to the extent that both ends are no longer attached. They have separated into two pieces. It is not necessary that it breaks into two pieces; it can break into several pieces. The fractures can be very painful, and there are reasons behind it. When the bone snaps, it often ruptures the soft tissues surrounding it, which causes a lot of pain to the injured person. Moreover, the body can also cause intense muscle spasms in order to hold the broken pieces of bones in place. Therefore, it is very crucial that one calms the injured person down and talks to them to relieve them of any stress.

Fractures can widely be categorized into two types: open fractures and closed fractures. Open fractures are often caused by heavy and energetic impacts. The broken bone penetrates through the skin and pushes out so that it is protruding, and it is visible to the naked eye. There is an open wound as a result, and there is the possibility for dirt and bacteria to enter and contaminate the wound, thus causing infection.

On the other hand, in a closed fracture, the bone has snapped but is still under the skin. In this case, a visible bulge is observed, which is the broken bone pushing against the surface of the skin. Both of these types of fractures can cause great inconvenience for the adventurer. Their mobility can be compromised to a great extent, and it will take a lot of time until the bone has completely healed. One should talk to the injured person and evaluate the injury by talking to them about the pain they may be experiencing. They should be prohibited from moving the injured area and should be given lots of water to drink. Moving a lot after an accident can possibly cause the nerve to damage and blood vessels to severe. As a result, one can bleed internally, and if a lot of blood is lost, then they can die.

Although it is usually very easy to identify a broken bone by the pain, deformed appearance, and the swelling that results from a fracture, it can sometimes be difficult to identify them. When a bone breaks, there is a snapping sound that is an indication of the broken bone. There is visible bruising and swelling around the injured area. Sometimes, there might not be a snapping sound but a grinding noise, which can also indicate a broken bone. Moreover, it might not hurt when the bone is stationary, but it can hurt when there is a movement of the injured area when you press the injured area or put weight on the injured area. The person might also feel dizzy and sick as a result of the sudden shock of a broken bone. Once you have successfully identified the break and the location of the injury, it is time to treat it. Due to the harsh impact, there might be wounds on the injury site, and one needs to tend to the resulting wounds. If there is bleeding, do not apply pressure. If a wound results from a bone break, applying hard pressure to the wound site can aggravate the damage done. Instead, one should press the pressure points.

As stated in the previous chapter, applying pressure to the arteries between the heart and the wound site can stop or significantly slow down the bleeding. After you have successfully stopped the bleeding, disinfect the wound after washing it with sterile water. You should bandage it if necessary and then proceed to address the fracture itself.

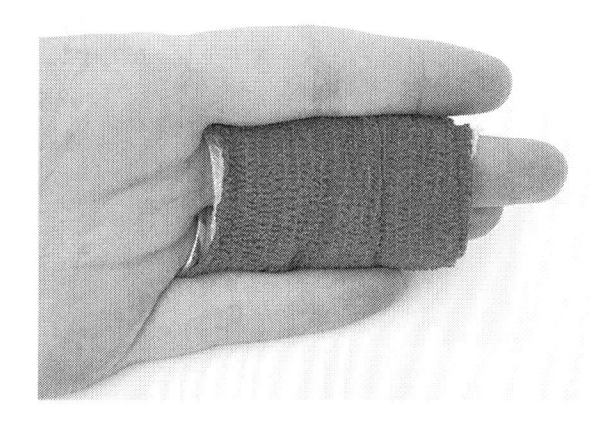

You now need to set the broken bone into its original anatomical position. This will relieve the injured person in a lot of pain. Medically this process is called applying traction. You need to hold the intact part of the limb in place and apply downward pressure to set the broken bone in its original place. Once the bone is in the correct position, it is time to splint it.

Making a Splint

The function of the splint is to immobilize the broken bone so that it does not cause any further damage or hurt the nerves or blood vessels. Since in the woods, it is difficult to find a commercially manufactured splint that is used for medical purposes, one needs to make a makeshift one. The best possible choice is a broken branch. Trees are usually everywhere, and it also allows one to make a reasonable splint. Take around half an inch thick branch and break it to be at least the size of the broken bone. Place one branch on either side of the broken bone and tie them together. Make sure you include the joint between the break, in order to effectively restrict any movement. So, for example, if there is a fracture in the lower arm, make sure you include the elbow when applying the splint. The splint should extend from the lower arm, past the joint, and to the upper arm. One can use gorilla tape, handkerchiefs, shoelaces, or even bandanas to tie the splints together. However, make sure that you do not tie it too tightly so that it cuts off the circulation of blood.

The purpose of applying a splint to the fracture is so that the bone is immobile when it is being transferred to the hospital. The rugged and rocky terrain outdoors can be dangerous for an un-splinted fracture while moving, and the broken bone can pierce through the skin due to the haphazard movement. To provide comfort to the injured person and to further limit any movement, it is advised that the splint should be padded. One can use any stuffing, including, but not limited to, blankets, clothing, and handkerchiefs. The injured person can assist with the bandaging and the splinting process.

In cases where, in particular, the thigh bones are injured, a traction splint has to be built and put on the injured person. It is a mechanical device that applies traction to the broken bone. It secures and immobilizes the upper and the lower leg and places a tension device at the foot. To make an improvised traction splint, one should use a branch to splint along the leg bone up to the armpit of the injured person. On the other side of the leg, the branch should expand to the groin area of the person. Both of these branches should be tied together like a normal splint. A stick should be attached across both the branches at the bottom- almost near the ankle. A wrap needs to be prepared; it can be a rope or a handkerchief or any similar material that will serve as an ankle wrap. One end of the ankle wrap is secured around the cross stick and the other tied to the ankle itself. A traction splint is now successfully constructed; however, to vary the tension in the mechanism, u can use a small stick to twist the ankle wrap and create tension. This last process will be similar to increasing pressure in a tourniquet.

Be mindful of the material you use to make a splint. It is not necessary that you use a piece of branch, you can use a metal rod, rolled up newspapers, long spoons, or rulers. Using a metal rod on a hot day is not advisable as the temperature can heat up the rod and cause great discomfort to the injured. If left in place and exposed to heat for a long period of time, it can burn the skin of the injured and expose them further to an infection.

Dislocations and Other Injuries

A joint is where two or more bones come together and meet. The dislocation is when this position, which causes the bones to move, is injured. The surrounding tendons, nerves, and muscles can also be injured due to a joint dislocation and cause further complications. One can identify a joint dislocation by the appearance of the joint - it will look deformed. Moreover, the person will experience intense pain, reduced muscle strength, and would have difficulty moving the joint. The main cause of such an injury is intense trauma or when someone falls on a certain joint. The pressure from the impact to the joint can cause the bones to become dislocated from their original position. Dislocation can cause the ligament that holds the bones in place to loosen or become injured, thus creating a possibility of a dislocation of the same site to become easier in the future.

If there is a wound as a result of the trauma, treat it as mentioned previously. To treat the dislocation itself, try to reset the bone into its original place. Medically this process is known as reduction. Use gentle maneuvers to help the bone into the position and take into consideration the discomfort it might cause to the injured. Depending on the swelling, give some pain killers to the injured and use appropriate force while setting the bone. It is easier to reset a dislocated knee cap, fingers, and toes. However, if the dislocation occurs at the high or the elbow tries to evacuate immediately and let a professional reset the bone back in its place. Wrong maneuvers to bring the bone back to its place can aggravate the injury further. After the bone has been reduced, the injured person will feel evident soreness and stiffness in the area around the injury. It is advised to apply a splint to the injury, just like a fracture, to limit the mobility of the limb and allow it to heal. If the dislocation is in the shoulder or the elbow, you can create a sling. A sling will allow you to hold your limb against your chest and allow you to hold it stationary.

Dislocations can occur at any joint site, including the knee, shoulder, toes, and fingers. However, the most common type of dislocation is observed at the shoulder. The shoulder bones are joined together in the sockets shaped like a ball. When dislocation of the shoulder occurs, the bones come out of these sockets. To reduce the bone, one needs to get this ball back into the socket. As stated before, injured muscles tend to spasm in order to hold the broken or dislocated bones into place. They become stiff over time, and therefore it is important that the bone is reduced as quickly as possible.

Shoulder Dislocation

To treat a shoulder dislocation, have the injured person lie down on the floor with their face upwards. Relax the patient by talking to them, and gradually guide their arm horizontally so that it is a 45-degree angle to their body. If there is any resistance, do not force any movement. Now pull the arm towards you so that the head of the dislocated bone has moved beyond the cup and slips right into the socket. If you need any support, place your leg on the victim's side, right under the armpit. This will allow you to exert additional pressure if need be. Another method that can be used to reduce a shoulder dislocation involves the rotation of the arm. This can be a little painful and can sometimes not work as efficiently. To perform this, one needs to lie their patient down on their back. While the person is lying down, gently rotate their forearm until the forearm is facing upwards. At this point, the hand should make the letter L but inverted, with the longer part being the forearm and the smaller being the upper arm going into the shoulder. Now further rotate the arm at the side so that the upper arm is right above the shoulder cap, and the lower arm is touching the head. The arm should still be making an L shape. If this does not work, it is advised to sling the arm and wait for emergency aid. Moreover, if the arm is resisting while performing this procedure, do not force it. Forcing can produce a toque capable of breaking a bone.

Muscle Cramps

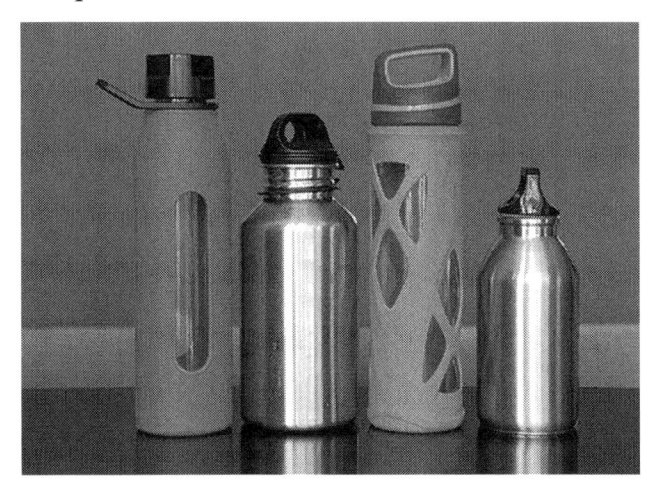

Muscle cramps are a strong and painful contraction of the muscles in the body. Muscles tighten during a cramp, and they can last from a few seconds to a couple of minutes. They are caused due to various reasons, but they are often caused by an injury or the overuse of a muscle, like excessive exercise. The likelihood of a cramp increase in cold weather or when a muscle is submerged in cold water. Dehydration can also cause muscle cramps, and in survival situations, when one does not have immediate access to water, the chances of experiencing a muscle cramp increase.

To treat a muscle cramp, stretch, and massage the muscle that is bothering you. A cold pack or heating pad can also help relieve the pain due to cramps. Use cold or hot water and fill it in the container to give a hot or cold bottle massage to the area. If one experiences cramps in the leg, they should walk around and jiggle their leg. Moreover, stretching the calf muscle can also bring some relief to the injured person. One can stretch their calf muscles by lying down flat and flexing their feet towards themselves.

Additional extensive and exhausting walks in the wilderness can often lead to sprains. The stretching or tearing of the ligament around the joints is known as sprains. It is caused when a trauma forces the joint to perform a movement beyond its capability. Most of the sprains are characterized by swelling and bruising, but it can be treated. Differentiating between a fracture and a sprain is important, and one can do that if they are aware of their symptoms.

Sprains

Sprains can cause swelling, bruises, limit movement, and cause difficulty while bearing weight. The main difference is that sprains cause muscle spasms and muscle weakness, while fractures are characterized by bone tenderness, especially when the injured site is made to bear weight. To treat a sprain, make sure you ice it. However, ice is not available in the woods; therefore, one can use cold water or snow and fill it in a container to be used as an ice pack. Moreover, make sure you give the injured area considerable rest and splint it if needed.

Although these injuries are treatable in a survival situation, it is extremely important that one tries not to incur them in the first place. Make sure that you are aware of the surroundings and do make any careless decisions. Every step is taken, and every move made needs to be cautious and calculated. If a slope looks too steep to walk down on, try to find an alternative route. If you feel exhausted and are hurting, make sure you take a quick break. Precaution is better than an injury in the woods, where help is uncertain.

Note: If you're in a life-threatening or emergency medical situation, seek medical assistance immediately.

Chapter 5

Food Poisoning and Choking

People usually do not take the same precautions in the woods that they might back home when it comes to food. At home, people are very cautious about how they store the food and worry about its hygiene, but in the woods, food is not readily available, and we do not abide by these food safety measures. Finding something to eat in the wild is sometimes the only goal of an adventurer, and hunger usually drives our decision making and not our minds. Due to this lack of safety measures, the food can cause an upset stomach and might even lead to death in some cases.

Imagine a scenario where you are in the wild and rummaging the forest for some kind of food to satiate your hunger. Finally, you come across some fish, and you clean it to the best of your abilities and eat it. However, several hours later, you start to feel sick. You realize you have food poisoning, what do you do in a situation? Or you eat the fish and choke on one of its very fine bones. You are gasping for air and choking on the bone. How do you tackle such a situation?

The chapter below explores the issue of food poisoning in a survival situation and also delves into the ways one should deal with a person who is choking on food. These situations can lead to death, and therefore it is important that one should be prepared to tackle them if they occur.

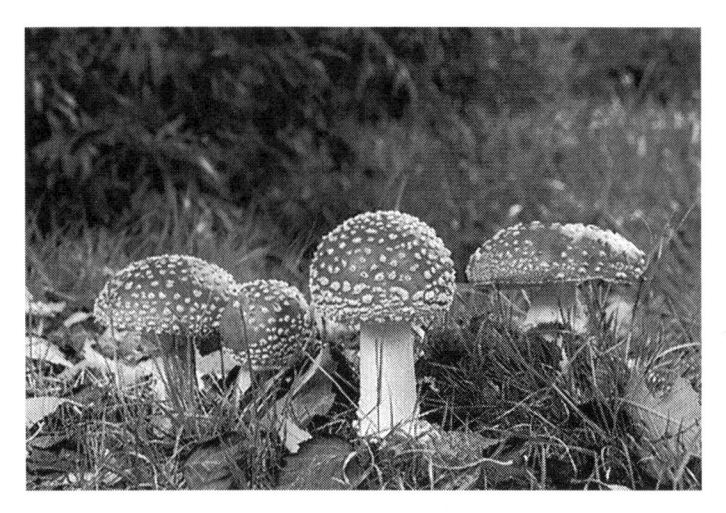

Poisonous Mushrooms

Food Poisoning

Food poisoning is an illness caused when one consumes food that has been contaminated by dangerous bacteria. It can also be caused by eating spoiled food and eating impure water, which is something that many campers do in the wild. Unpasteurized milk, undercooked meat, contaminated and cross-contaminated food are the most common sources of food poisoning. E Coli and Salmonella are some of the most common types of bacteria that can cause food poisoning.

To prevent your food from being contaminated by the likes of such viruses, it is important that food is cooked and stored properly. Some of the symptoms that one experiences during food poisoning include nausea, vomiting, headaches, stomach cramps, and diarrhea. These symptoms can occur almost instantly or may occur after a few days. With proper treatment, these symptoms will go away in a couple of days, but in some severe cases, they can last up to a week. The bacteria produce toxins, which are the real threat to a person, not the bacteria itself. Moreover, sometimes naturally occurring poisons and toxins in certain plants, fish, or mushrooms can also lead to food poisoning.

Proper Food Storage

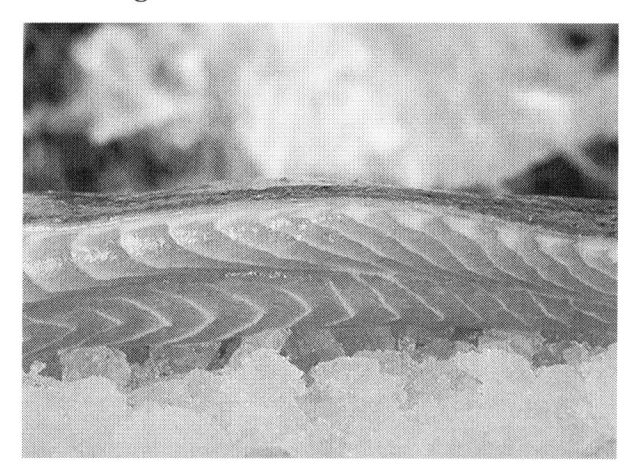

Foods like fish, meat, and dairy products are more likely to be contaminated than other kinds of food. They provide an environment in which bacteria can thrive and can produce toxins. However, the risk of contamination can be greatly reduced if these foods are cooked and stored properly. Adventurers often make the mistake of carrying meat with them to trip, and they do not take measures to refrigerate them properly. The harmful microorganisms in the meat duplicate and make it dangerous. Even if the meat is cooked thoroughly, putting it in the same container can cause it to cross-contaminate because of the harmful fluid that was left behind in the container from the raw meat. This is one of the common mistakes that is witnessed amongst explorers. If one takes precaution to control the temperature and have proper storage for the food, the probability of food poisoning can be greatly reduced. If someone wishes to carry meat or any other food that requires to be stored at a preferable temperature, they should do so in a thermal container or cooler. These will keep the food hot or cold and prevent it from going bad. Moreover, one can use a blanket to cover their cooler to increase its effectiveness in keeping the food hot or cold as it would protect it from the sunlight. Moreover, it is very important that one washes their hands with soap before preparing their food, smoking, and using the toilet. If soap is not available, rather than ignoring this process, one should use any source of sterile water to rinse their hands.

During food poisoning, people tend to throw-up a lot, and they lose a lot of water content from their bodies. This leads to dehydration, which, on its own, can cause many problems. That is why one should drink a lot of water during food poisoning to restore the electrolytes and the water content. It is recommended that one liter of water should be mixed with one teaspoon of salt and four teaspoons of sugar to rehydrate oneself.

Additionally, one should avoid preparing food for others until a few days after their symptoms have stopped. This is to avoid spreading any germs to people in their company. One should also avoid eating solid foods at first as they might throw up and take everything in fluid form. They should take as many fluids as they think they can without feeling sick. Once they start to feel better, they should switch to solid, soft foods like bananas. Also, fatty foods should be avoided as the body is not in a state to digest fat during food poisoning.

One should pack antibacterial tablets in the first aid kit and have them during food poisoning to counter any bacteria that might be causing the symptoms. Ginger and apple cider vinegar is also said to have properties that can help during food poisoning.

Choking

Choking is when a piece of food or any small object is stuck in the airway and prevents one from breathing. Choking on food usually occurs due to people drinking and eating too rapidly. The threat posed by choking is minimal and short-lived; however, if one does not know what to do when someone is choking on something, it can also lead to death.

One can tell if someone is choking when they suddenly start coughing aggressively and have trouble breathing. The food is cutting their air supply and needs to be forced out of the system for them to breathe. A person who is choking on food may also be unable to speak properly or make any noise. Moreover, due to the lack of oxygen, their lips and their nails might start to turn blue, indicating that they are not able to breathe. One should put both their hands on the neck to indicate to other people that they are choking so that they can be helped.

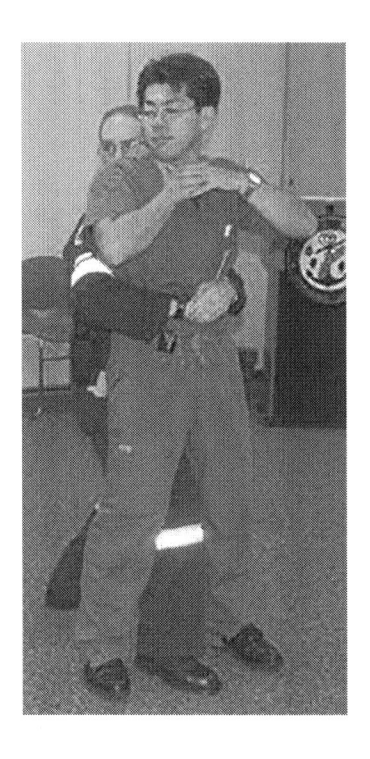

The American Red Cross recommends the use of the "five and five" method to help a person who is choking. This method calls for the person who is helping to use the heel of their hand to hit the choking person five times between their shoulder blades. However, this technique should not be employed if the person choking is a child.

After performing this method, the Heimlich maneuver should be practiced on the person choking. To perform a Heimlich maneuver, the person carrying out this technique should position themselves behind the choking person. Then they should proceed to wrap both their hands around the choking person's waist, before placing one of their hands, closed in a fist, over the choking person's abdominal region- right above their navel. The freehand should be used to grip the fist to thrust them in an upward motion. This motion should be repeated five times, and the Heimlich maneuver should be alternatively performed with the "five and five" technique until the object obstructing the airway is pushed out.

In the case of the baby, sandwich his body between your hands. Providing good support to the head and the jaw applies pressure on the chest, or on the abdomen in case of a larger infant, to push the obstruction. Once you see the obstructing material emerging from the throat, remove it with your fingers.

CPR

If the person is having trouble breathing, call for help!

Then CPR should be performed immediately.

This important technique should be learned by every individual, as it can come in handy anytime and anywhere. To perform CPR, the person should be made to lie down flat on the back on a plain surface. The person carrying the procedure out should kneel on their side and place their hand on the middle of their chest, with one hand placed over another. Once you have placed your hand properly, push down on the person's chest to mimic a chest compression.

You need to be quick and achieve almost a hundred compressions in a minute. Remember that this should be employed only as a last choice when the person is not breathing and not responding. Performing this method requires strength and can get aggressive. You might break the person's ribs, but you have to do what it takes to save a life.

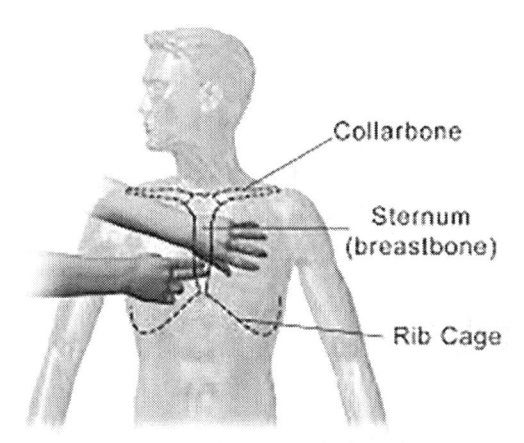

Locate the Sternum

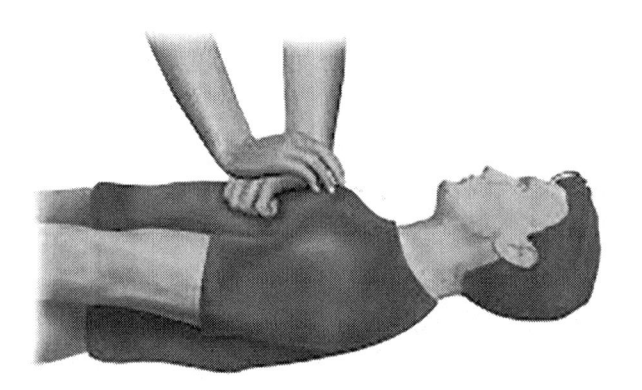

Position Hands Over Sternum

Moreover, as stated before, one should avoid eating any unfamiliar plants as they might cause an allergic reaction, which can result in the inflammation of the windpipe and thus choking.

Even though the rest of the book has encouraged traveling alone, such situations may arise where the help of another person is required, and at times self-healing is not possible. If you are a new explorer that it is advisable that you stick close to the trails made out in the maps of the areas you visit where it is likely that other explorers can be easily found. Otherwise, explorers have to be very careful when exploring on their own since it is a very dangerous craft. Initially, group explorers can be administered, and then once new explorers become seasoned explorers, they can tackle the wild on their own along with the help of these self-healing tips.

Note: If you're in a life-threatening or emergency medical situation, seek medical assistance immediately.

Chapter 6

Emotional and Spiritual Healing in the Wilderness

"Green Day," a famous American rock band, once used the words "information nation" in their record-breaking song called "American Idiot." The lyrics of this song perfectly describe the situation of many people and nations in the world. These days, people and governments are information-oriented, with eyes glued to some kind of a screen at all times of the day. This roots out all other activities in the day, and the extent of the issue reaches many households as well. The issue takes route in the personal lives of people and then develops throughout all aspects of their lives. So much so that having a meal without watching something or scrolling through social media feeds is nonexistent, pretty much anywhere in the world.

Throughout the spreading of this global phenomenon, experts in the fields of psychology and mental health have been talking about the adverse effects of technology on the untrained human minds. However, this issue has been taken lightly since the global technology takeover shows no signs of slowing down or stopping any time soon. Many of our personal places have been invaded by screens and other such hysteria that our unconditioned minds have had no time to adapt to the new world. This has taken away our "alone time," resulting in a mental lapse that has given birth to a fragile future generation that is overdependent on technology for all of their problems.

In such times the only alone time that a person can get is a vacation; however, that too has been crowded out by phones, laptops, and cameras that work together to spoil the moment. Wilderness exploration, however, is the only activity left to heal the brain from the worries of the world. This chapter focuses on the many different takes on mental health in the modern world and how beneficial the wilderness is for spiritual and mental healing. This is a different form of "self-healing" that has not been explored in this resource up till now. Nonetheless, it is still a form of self-healing and is important in sustaining happier lifestyles. The main focus of the two sections in this chapter is to analyze how the wilderness works to relieve the mind of any pent-up stress. Through the analysis, readers may get a good grip on how the brain works in the crowded urban life and the wilderness.

Through the two sections below, the readers must also learn to appreciate the wilderness. The wilderness has magical healing abilities that no other place on this Earth has. Be it trekking, hiking, fishing, camping, or any other wilderness related activity, research shows that the amount of mental relief received from such activities is greater than urban activities such as watching your favorite sports game or playing a video game to pass the time. Once explorers experience these magical abilities for themselves, the appreciation will follow on their own.

Several research studies and personal accounts have been used up to make the following two sections possible. The amount of effort in the research shows how this phenomenon is very real and needs to be talked on more. Hopefully, this section gives readers more confidence to explain to other people about how the wilderness is a magical self-healing place, second to none. The purpose of this research is to give concrete evidence to support the claims brought about by personal experiences of self-healing and mental/spiritual healing in the wilderness. The sources used for evidence in this chapter are trustworthy, and the personal experiences are verified by fellow explorers to ensure that the truest form of wilderness is represented in this book. Any made-up sources were deemed illegible, and therefore, were not taken into account for the analysis in the following chapters.

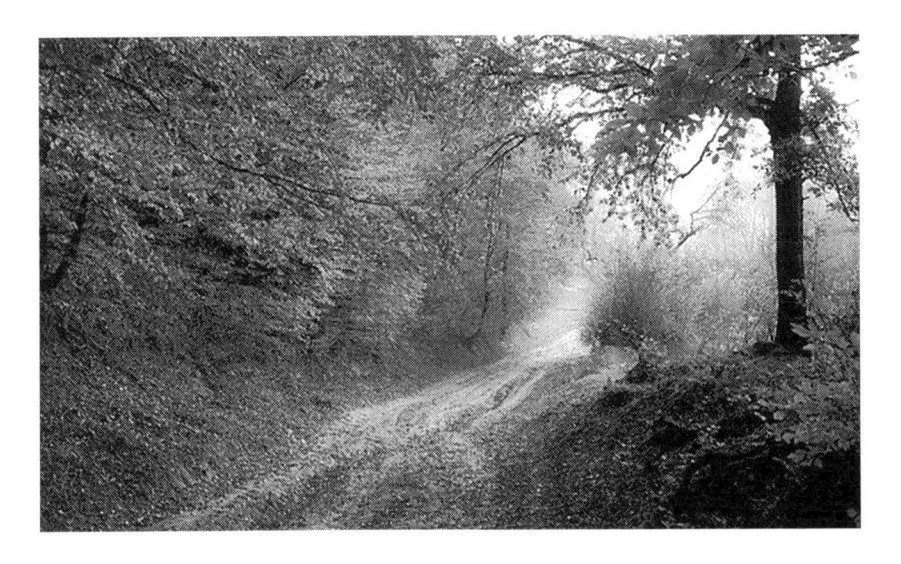

Silent Therapy

Being alone is different from being lonely! This section has been designed to convey this thought in an effective manner so that individuals and explorers' sort through their feelings in an organized manner. In the past few years, being alone has been confused for being lonely. With the advent of smartphones, we are never alone, and that is a concerning fact! Before the inception of the technological age (21st century), there were always times when individuals had some time to catch up with their surroundings. They always had time to take a moment from their work to observe and take energy from their surroundings. Their minds were always aware of what was going around them. As compared to the modern generation, there are stark differences. Because of the notion of never being alone (by having a smartphone), the mind is not as alert as it once was. Those moments that were used to take in the surroundings and to sharpen the mind have now been replaced with individuals flicking through their phone screens to catch up with their friends or to play a game.

The main takeaway from these facts is that our leisure time has now been taken over by a schedule-less, chaotic, screen spending activities. Instead of relieving stress, as a leisure activity should, such activities only build on the trauma by conveying riveting storylines based on fictional events by labeling them as thrillers.

Explorers are at a benefit in these circumstances since they can access the most surreal parts of the world where there is no electricity or a cell phone signal that can divert your attention. Studies have shown that since the '90s, there has been an increase in wilderness exploration and therapy programs throughout the United States. The participants in these programs reported that alone time in nature caused them to reflect on their lives in a much deeper setting than any other place they could envisage. The end results of such programs also illustrated a roadmap for explorers of the future. The results indicated that the wilderness is key to spending some alone time as it is vital to relieving stress and restoring attention. The first one of these two results is explained in this section while the other is explained in the next section.

The silence that is experienced in the wild is a very thought-provoking experience that has a strange and magical effect on the brains of explorers. The entire process of this silent therapy leads to the end results that were found in many wilderness programs. The first time that an explorer goes into the wild, there are a few things that may not seem certain. The first few days alone in the wild, an explorer experiences a period of solitude.

This is a well-researched phenomenon that shows the transition between life in urban cities and traveling along through the forest as the noise from the insects forms a constant base at the back of your mind rather than the city noises that overpower the mind. This period of solitude has been described as a very vital part of the trip where the explorer re-examines his life decisions, his relation to nature, and his relation to God. This period has been described as mentally enriching and spiritually freeing. (Daniel, 2018).

Solitude

For this section, we will refer to it as the "solitude period." This period lasts for around one to three days. So, why does something like this exist, and why is it so important? To put it simply, this period exists because the mind is not as fast to adapt to changes as the mind it. If an explorer moves from the comfort and hustle-bustle of the city to the quiet wilderness, then it takes some time for the mind to adjust to the sudden change in setting. It is the micro-level changes that make the difference, like the rapid chirping and hooting that takes place in the wilderness that brings the spirit closer to the natural element. The mind also needs time to comprehend the level of comfort that has suddenly changed. With that comes an internal conflict as to the purpose of wilderness exploration. However, after being forced to spend some time in this solitude period, the mind questions the rapid technological advancements that the human civilization has made. This mainly happens because of the peace the mind experiences that seemed unreal in the "real world."

The first three days of any trek, camping trip, a hiking trip, or any backpacking trip is hard, emotionally. This happens due to, as explained earlier, the drastic change of lifestyle. However, it is important to understand that, along with the emotional responses, the physical responses are also responsible for this period of solitude to exist. The physical output of individuals generally increases more than twice of what they did back in their urban lifestyles. Due to this added strain on the brain, the period is an emotionally important one.

Once exhausted physically, the emotional wit of an individual is tested. So, in simple terms, the physical aspect of the trip is why this period of solitude comes into existence. This correlation is important to note, in order to understand why the brain forces an individual to ask questions of existence and life.

Another aspect of this silent therapy and period of solitude is the small nuances that force the mind to react differently. For example, the air that you breathe in the wilderness is very different from the urban air. Something as small as breathing is different, so the bigger things will have a much different impact on the brain. Coupled with these small differences in the physical stress, which then causes the emotional stress to be stripped down so that the individual can find answers to some key questions that life has dealt them.

The silent therapy provides relief from the "race" that goes on in city life. This relief allows a lot of time for reflection, which increases trust in nature and the being that created it all. The peace present within the wilderness is somewhat transcended into the explorer's mind.

In order to live a life without uncertainty, a life with a clear state of mind, then it is recommended that such changes of self-reflection are never ignored. Self-reflection is an important element that was crowded out by the technological advancements spoken about at the start of this chapter. The benefits of this self-reflection are explained in the next section following a life in the wilderness after the period of solitude has ended. The end is marked by a mental revival, and individuals are usually observed to be more mentally present and available! More of this mental revival has been explained below; however, for that to be achieved, a period of solitude has to happen!

The Mental Revival

The second part of this chapter focuses on the emotional and spiritual enlightenment that the individual experiences after the period of solitude end. This is the self-healing part of this chapter and shows how an individual can be emotionally rejuvenated in the wilderness. National Geographic and other such institutions have conducted vast experiments on how the wilderness can benefit the mental state of individuals. Such studies and their results have been analyzed to give a summary of how this metal revival takes place.

After the first few days, the brain has had enough time to recalibrate according to its new surroundings. The emotional connection to nature helps in allowing the brain to recalibrate to the surroundings. The brain is now in perfect tune with the surroundings. Studies have found that individuals can smell, hear, and see better within the first few days of being in the wild. This, of course, is the result of the mental rejuvenation that has taken place over the period of solitude.

National Geographic conducted one such experiment that took individuals into the wilderness and measured their brain activity by measuring their brain waves (Williams, 2020). The end results showed compared the brain wave activity of individuals in the wild with two groups who remained in the city. The results went on to support the thesis that the mental state of individuals in the wild was in a better condition than those who remained in the city.

Not only that, but the test also showed that the brain (pre-frontal cortex to be more specific) showed less activity when the individuals were in the wild. This means that the brain, when in the thick of an urban city, is usually overworked and stressed. This requires the brain to remain in a hyper state and is never switched off. The time off, in the wilderness, allows individuals to take some time off and recalibrate. The break allows individuals to become more in tune with the Earth and to relax their brain for a while.

It is a well-known fact that people living near green spaces for most of their lives are less likely to report any mental fatigue or stress than people who do not have such privilege. This fact, coupled with the analysis of the reduced brain activity shows that an individual has the ability to relax him/herself in the wild. While in their regular life, this privilege is not accessible since the human advancements act as a hindrance towards achieving mental peace.

Along with the third or the fourth day of the wilderness trip, the brain's ability to recall things becomes better and is related to the cognitive recall. The relaxed state of the brain allows for it to function more efficiently, allowing an individual to smell, see, hear, and recall things at a more natural pace. It's like a person who has just received a great massage, and his body is as good as new. Well, it is kind of like a massage, but for your brain!

The most important aspect of a wilderness trip is yet to be explored in this section. Perhaps the most prominent change seen in an individual on a wilderness trip is in his/her way of thinking. Nature can be inspiring, and just as it is rejuvenating for the mind, it can rejuvenate the spirit as well! Nature can motivate an induvial to think differently and view scenarios in their life with a different perspective than they would have initially done. This motivational activity is a result of the period of solitude, where the explorer is forced to look at their situation through different perspectives. They can then apply the same phenomenon to different aspects of their lives to comprehend it better.

The inspirational qualities of the wilderness come from the surreal beauty that can be surprising for first-time explorers. The natural wonders can make individuals think about their perspectives (and change them) and rethink their ideas on life. Such inspirational moments can also help creators and writers move through a mental block.

A mental block is a creator's puzzle that arises when they seem to have no new ideas to work on. Exploring nature can give writers, artists, and sculptors different ideas on how to interpret life in their next projects. This is the main reason why creators (considered as free spirits) are often seen encouraging other people to explore the world. It is because they truly have free spirits, freer than most people who have never visited the wilderness. "Beauty evokes creation," which is the main take away for the spirit from this experience.

Wilderness Meditation

Another spiritual benefit of the wilderness is that it is the perfect place for meditators. The silence and the surreal beauty of the place that an explorer is it takes its effect on the explorer's mind. An explorer who also practices meditation can benefit greatly from this characteristic of the wild. Many explorers tend to plan their trips for the sole purpose of meditating in the wild because of the surreal experience that it usually tends to be. The weather that surrounds explorers and the fact that no one else is around to disturb them is a good prerequisite for carrying out their mediating activities in the wild.

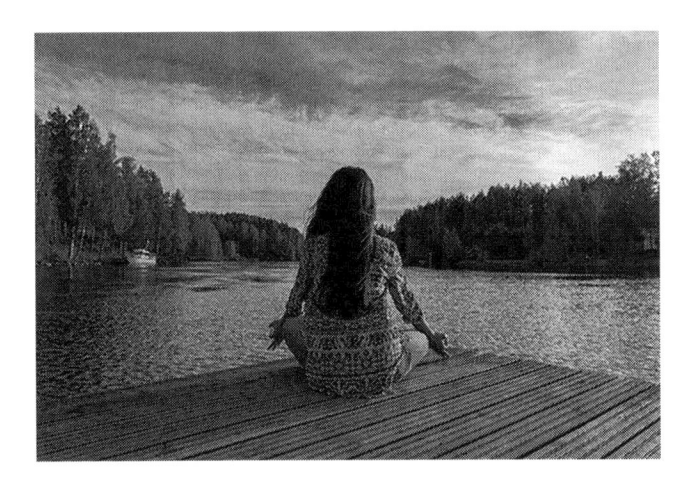

Meditation is another way to cleanse the soul off of the external stress so that the mind can gain clarity. This is more of an active way for spiritual self-healing, whereas silent therapy was a passive act by the wilderness on the explorer mind. Explaining meditation in this chapter would be deviating from the topic of how the wilderness is a self-healer since meditations is a vast topic. Meditation involves a guided path and an unguided path that will be well suited for other experts; however, it is mentioned here since it is a viable option to actively self-heal in the wild.

Along with gaining physical fitness, the mental fitness of individuals is also tested in the wilderness. Usually, the test creates a better person who is more emotionally and spiritually mature. There have not been many scientific studies based on the phenomenon because it is so difficult to quantitate. The happiness factor cannot just be given a number; however, how you feel when you complete your wilderness experience is what matters the most. Maybe the true magic of nature is to be hidden from scientists forever, but the magical feeling is not hidden from the explorers!

Chapter 7

Altitude Sickness

Some of the best views of the landscape can be seen from a higher point (height-wise) in the area. However, there are many people that are not able to climb/trek to a higher place because of the physical limitations presented by the conditions that an unexperienced explorer cannot overcome. This chapter focuses on tips and techniques to help explorers deal with the sickness that comes with height, called altitude sickness. Another name for altitude sickness is called mountain sickness. This is a normal condition that can be overcome by explorers if they train their bodies according to the techniques given below.

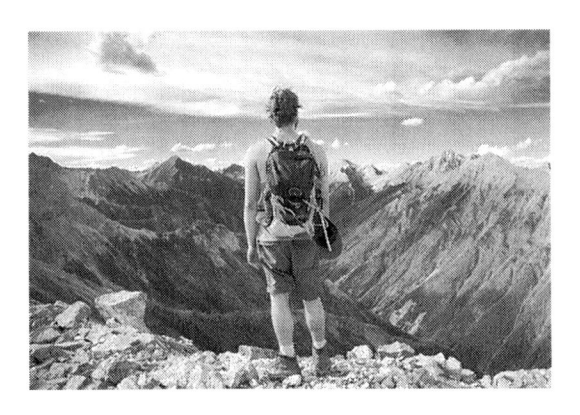

Altitude sickness is basically a number of symptoms that strike a person when they gain height (altitude) rapidly. So rapidly, that their body is no acclimatized to it and reacts in a negative way. The science behind this is very simple! As a person climbs higher, the pressure drops to lower than what they are used to. This lower pressure results in lower availability of oxygen. The body needs time to get used to the different conditions that it is in; thus, the body needs to be trained with lower gains in height rather than sudden height changes. This case is similar to when a person goes to dive, and if he rapidly gains depth, then the body can be crushed by the immense pressure exerted by the water that the lungs cannot cope with on their own. Even at lower depth gains a diving tank is necessary.

The symptoms of this condition are mild headaches, nausea, dizziness, vomiting, and lack of sleep (problems while sleeping). The last symptom is caused by another common symptom of the illness, which is shortness of breath. Naturally, if less oxygen is available, then the body will get tired at a faster rate since it is working harder to survive. This situation covers the shortness of breath symptom that is the very first sign observed after nausea and dizziness. Another pointer about this sickness is that it may be observed after a few hours of the height change or even immediately. Loss of appetite is also a common symptom in some cases. The person may not eat enough and try to soldier through the sickness; however, this is one of the first signs to figuring out what is wrong and treating it.

One important thing to grasp before moving on to the self-healing part of the chapter is the incidence of the sickness. Altitude sickness is very common and can happen to anyone! Even professional athletes get it. However, ignoring it and soldiering on with it can prove to be fatal since two severe kinds of altitude sicknesses are High Altitude Pulmonary Edema (HACE) and High Altitude Cerebral Edema (HACE). These two types refer to the fluid being built up in the lungs and in the brain, respectively. These two are the most severe form of altitude sickness and have proven to be deadly on several occasions. Even though these are very rare cases, they can still appear in any situation, which is why the procedures and prevention tips explained below should be taken seriously.

Self-Healing from Altitude Sickness

A good omen with this sickness is that it may reduce with time as the body learns to adapt to the new surroundings. However, there are a few self-healing tips that can be administered to help with the process. The main thing that has to be the attention of the victim/explorer is to quicken the process acclimatization. The faster the body adapts to the surroundings, the faster the symptoms of the sickness will disappear.

If you get a couple of symptoms together, then it may be better to take quick action. If the change in altitude was profound (couple hundred feet in a small amount of time), then you may have altitude sickness. Knowing this makes it easier to treat since acknowledging it is the first step. Ignoring it would lead to nowhere! The best solution to altitude sickness is to reduce the altitude. This is the best solution since the rapid decline in height is going to take the body back to an environment that it is used to. The lower altitude must be lower than 4000 feet, at the very least.

If you are a new explorer/trekker and the feeling of this sickness is too much to handle, then it may be a good idea to reduce your elevation as soon as possible. However, if they are very mild symptoms and you can carry on, then some medication can be administered to help ease up the symptoms and get the body acclimatized at a faster rate.

Ibuprofen is the most common drug used in such situations. It can be found very easily in many drug stores across the world. Explorers instinctively carry such drugs with themselves as they can be very handy in drastic situations like the one being explored in this chapter. This drug can help with mild symptoms such as the headache and nausea that can prevent explorers from making integral decisions in the wild.

Another common drug that can help with the process of acclimatization is Acetazolamide. This is a common, over the shelf, drug that helps with respiration. This stimulant helps the body work more and metabolize oxygen at a higher rate. This process helps the body get used to the newer conditions at a faster rate. It can be administered when an individual is facing mild symptoms and needs a helping hand to get through the sickness. However, any worsening in his condition needs rapid action.

The first step of acknowledging the condition is important as explorers need to draw the line on when to push the body and when to stop. Any worsening needs to see a rapid drop in the altitude. The drop is hopefully going to fix things as smart explorers are going to take this decision before anything severe takes place.

In some cases, a portable oxygen chamber can also be taken. This chamber allows the traveler to carry air to higher conditions. In severe conditions, with a lack of oxygen, they can inflate this bag to maintain their body's oxygen levels and fight through the trek without getting the symptoms of altitudes sickness. This may be a common part of some trekker's high altitude gear. It can be stored in the backpack; however, it takes up space, which is necessary for some essentials.

In cases of unusually severe headaches and respiratory trouble, the explorer may be risking HACE and HAPE. In such cases, the explorer would need supplemental oxygen and some specific types of steroids that only doctors can administer. In such cases, the explorer must take quick action and descend. The descent is going to ease up the milder symptoms; however, the medication and treatment for HAPE and HACE must still be administered.

Some quick action techniques were communicated in this chapter for treating the conditions; however, it would be better if the explorers tried to prevent the sickness altogether. Some vital prevention techniques are communicated in the next section.

Tips on How to Prevent Altitude Sickness

A major prevention tip is to go slowly. There are many experts that will tell you that it is possible not to get altitude sickness at all. The proper technique to not get sick while going higher is to acclimatize the body with newer surroundings. The easiest way to do this is to climb slowly. Experts suggest that climbing a few thousand feet daily and then resting each day is the best way to complete a trek that experiences altitude changes of more than 10000 feet. The best way to tackle altitude changes is to get there gradually. Sure, it will take up more time; however, it will allow the body to adapt naturally rather than to take any drugs or administer supplemental oxygen. Along with resting a day for every 20000-3000 feet climb, experts suggest going slowly. Going slowly allows the individual to take deep breaths that will increase the oxygen in the red blood cell flow to different parts of the body.

Along with going slower, another common tip suggested by experts is to sleep lower. Experts suggest that even if you climb 1000 feet in a day, keep an option to sleep at a lower altitude. They suggest that climbing up in a day and then coming back down is not likely to cause altitude sickness since the body will not get time to react to the height change.

Sleeping in a lower area will solve any symptoms related to sleep that is caused by altitude sickness. This rule is even more valuable when the explorers are at a higher position. This will allow the body to cope with oxygen changes at the higher place in a more organized way, by allowing the relief of sleeping at a lower position. This process helps in acclimatizing the body with the new conditions.

Another prevention tip that has proved to be valuable for a lot of explorers is to drink a lot of water. It is advised that during the climbing trip, an individual should drink up to five liters of water each day. This may seem to be an easy task in hotter climates, but that is usually not the case in higher places. Even though it may seem tough to drink that much water in a colder area, it will still be very helpful. The body has to do extra work and requires a lot of oxygen, however since it is not getting enough oxygen from the surroundings, it needs extra water.

In addition, make sure that more than 60% of the calories that explorers are getting should be from carbohydrates. These carbohydrates are readily available energy sources that do not need a lot of breaking down by the body. This is beneficial in two ways. Firstly, the body will require a lot of energy for the climb, and these carbohydrates will readily provide that. The second benefit of doing this is to allow the body to focus more on the respiratory system rather than on the digestive system since carbohydrates do not need a lot of effort to be broken down into energy as compared to proteins and fats. So, it makes sure to drink a lot of water and eat right.

The most obvious tip in this section will be to avoid very drastic height changes in a single day. It is recommended to avoid climbing more than 1500 feet in a day as you should give appropriate time for your body to adjust since it is not about the physical condition of the explorer, as explained earlier. Altitude sickness does not depend on the physical condition; however, some people may react to it differently than others.

Even though all of the above-mentioned tips may help, the most important thing is to be able to judge the conditions on your own. A smart explorer is the one that takes quick action and decisions based on the conditions that nature has dealt with him/her. The most important tip is to be able to judge one's own body and determine whether the symptoms are there or not. If the symptoms are being ignored, then it is a bad decision to continue. Following the tips that have been talked about, the safest decision would be to halt the climb and return to the bottom if any member of the group feels nauseous or is exhibiting any other symptoms of altitude sickness.

Having said that, the most important thing is to have fun during a hike as it can be one of the most fulfilling experiences of your life. As explained in the previous chapter, beauty can evoke creativity from some of the deepest parts of your mind as you go on to explore some of the highest parts of the world.

Do not forget to rest after every few hours of climbing. The rest is not only so that the body can catch up with the surroundings but also for the spiritual and mental rejuvenation of explorers. Be sure to take full advantage of the view during the rest and rivet in some of the most peaceful locations that this Earth has to offer.

Chapter 8

The Backpack

Going on a trek or a hiking adventure is one of the best experiences that life has to offer. Only a few things can exceed the experience; however, there are a few things that can add to the experience. Packing the right gear in the most efficient manner possible is one of those things that can elevate your hiking experience to a whole new level!

The following chapter is based entirely on the backpack for the essentials that need to be packed for the trip. Explorers take their backpack everywhere; thus, it is necessary to add this chapter at the end since it is going to be the most informative one.

There are a few things that need to be planned way ahead of the trip in order to pack the most useful gear. An exploration trip needs to be well thought out since it revolves around the unpredictability of nature. Explorers need to prepare for every possibility out there, and so the planning phase takes a lot of time. Extra thought has to be given to the length of the trip since a lengthier trip is going to increase the number of items explorers bring along in their backpacks. This is essentially going to increase the weight of the bags and may cause some problems.. Exploration trips should be kept shorter since there are other factors associated with the length of the trip.

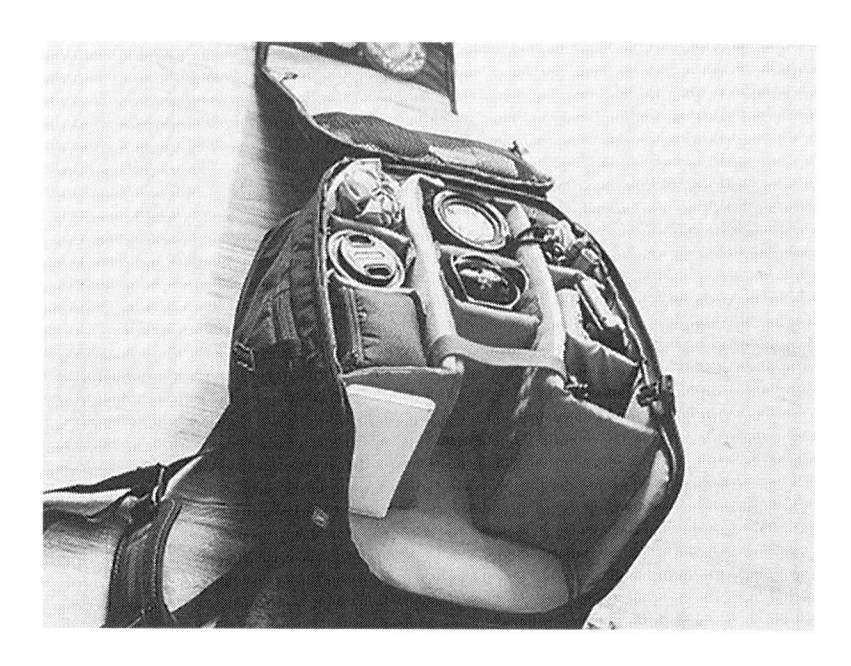

As mentioned earlier, the unpredictability of nature plays a vital role in the planning phase. The length of the trip may determine the type of weather that the explorer is going to face while on the trip! A shorter trip is going to require the explorer to face one kind of weather, whereas a longer trip may require the explorer to pack a lot of gear necessary to survive through different phases of the weather. Because of the technological advancements of the world, an explorer can plan their trip very efficiently. Through various sources, the forecast for the next few weeks can easily be charted out and the supplies that need to be stored can then be figured out as well.

Packing Options

With that being said, the first thing that an explorer should look for is a nice backpack that fits their needs. There are many backpacks available in the wilderness exploration market that cater to many needs. Some carry more weight while some are weatherproof. This should be a one-time investment, so choose something that you can use on many trips rather than for one specific trip only. A large backpack that holds around 60-100 lbs. These backpacks are designed to hold all of this stuff without overburdening the carrier. The newer technologies have made it possible for manufacturers to make bags that have built-in back and shoulder supports. The backpack selection is an essential part of the planning process as it may be a cause of fatigue during the trip. Fatigue may tarnish the overall experience of the wilderness trip.

Keeping in line with the theme, the first part of this chapter will cover all the essentials required to self-heal in the wild. All of these essentials were discussed in some shape or form in the other chapters. This is the final checklist for explorers so that any essential item is not missed out on. The rest of this chapter will focus on the other essentials necessary for survival in the wild. Without these items, a trekking/hiking/exploration trip is incomplete, and so it was necessary to include this checklist as well!

Self-Healing Essentials

The first and most important self-healing tool is the emergency kit, also called the first aid kit. Buy, or make the first aid kit that is going to travel with you at all times. Be sure to keep it in such a place in the backpack that it is accessible at all times. Because of the various situations that can arise in the wild, it is important to make the kit accessible at all times. The kits should also not weigh a lot since it would be a traveling kit. Some of the essential things to be kept in this kit are discussed below.

Medical Supplies

Plasters and Gauze dressing in various sizes should be kept in the first aid kit. Wounds are the most common aspect of the wild that will require constant attention. Keeping these dressing items means that explorers are well prepared to tackle the small cuts and bruises that are bound to take place in the wild. Along with plasters and dressings, safety pins, a pair of scissors, and some sterile gloves must also be kept in order to fully cater to all sorts of wounds, cuts, and other such problems that arise with wilderness exploration. Some sticky tape is also necessary to hold everything together. Make sure to get the surgical grade in order to have the most effective tool at your disposal. Experts also suggest keeping clean syringes in this section as they are useful in cleaning up and dressing wounds.

Talking about cleaning wounds, some disinfectant is key to survival in the wild. Use it wisely when dressing wounds as an infection in the wild can become a huge problem. The pain from a small wound would eventually become cumbersome and would need other medicines that are not available in the first aid kit.

The next part of this first aid kit addresses all types of animal and insect bites that were discussed in the first few chapters. To address such situations, explorers would need some alcohol-free cleansing wipes, a pair of fine-tipped tweezers, an antiseptic cream, and some distilled water to clean the wounds. The effective use of all of the above has been described in the first chapter. It is important to keep these items with the wound cleaning items as they may also come in handy when treating snake bites and spider bites.

A mechanical suction tool should also be kept along with this section as it is going to be useful if explorers are to visit parts that are notorious for snakes and spiders. These mechanical tools can help suck out the poison from the wound without the responders having to come in contact with the poison.

Bee stings were also discussed in the section of insect bites and stings, and so a bee sting kit can also be a useful tool. This is an optional tool as the treatment method has already been discussed that uses the materials from a normal first aid kit. However, someone that is allergic to bees/wasps will need this kit as it has useful drugs to treat the allergies that can become very agitating throughout the journey.

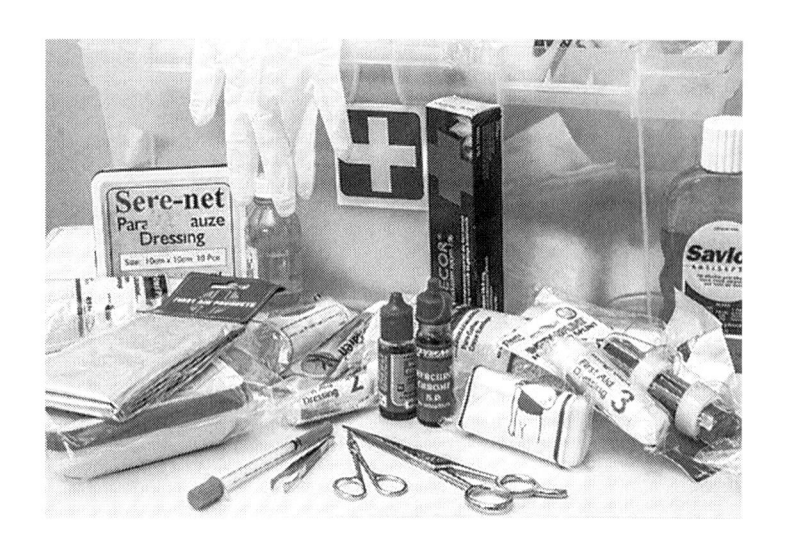

Medication

The next part of this medical kit is focused on the types of drugs that should be kept in it. The most common drugs that were discussed in the chapters were paracetamol and ibuprofen. These two are essential to relieve mild symptoms of many of the conditions that were discussed. Ibuprofen can even be used to treat some mild conditions of altitude sickness.

Anti-itching creams should also be kept just in case the insects get unbearable. The creams can help restrain the feeling of scratching up wounds again and again. Some antihistamines should also be kept in order to counter any allergic reactions. The value of antihistamines was also discussed in the insect bites chapter, where they become essential drugs to treat some symptoms of bug/snake bites.

The last part of the drug section includes simple cough medicine. Cough is also a common issue everywhere in the world and could be a sign of an allergic reaction to something in nature. Keeping a simple cough medicine is going to help manage the cough.

Fire Starters

It would be wise to keep a fire starter and some fuel for an emergency fire. An emergency fire may be something that is urgently required and could be delayed if explorers do not have the convenience of a fire starter at their disposal. This tool would help start a fire without going through the process of building a fire and keeping it going. However, explorers need to learn about not relying on the tool completely and should know proper fire-starting techniques as well. This tool should only be kept for emergency purposes.

Shelter

An emergency shelter must also be kept in the backpack since a need to spend the night at an emergency set up may arise. Usually, if explorers wander too far away from the base camp, then the emergency shelter comes in use. This shelter is quickly set up and is easily packed. The portability rating on such shelters is very high, allowing for quick and easy transportation. Only use it if the situation demands and it and do not make this shelter the primary shelter that you will be bringing on the trip. As the second section of this chapter explains the dynamics of a primary shelter. The secondary shelter is to help prevent the explorer from any external threats in a situation where the primary shelter is not accessible.

Hygiene

Health essentials are necessary, too, on any wilderness exploration trip! These products include hand sanitizers, soaps, sanitary towels, and menstrual products. Without these products, the self-healing is difficult since the hygiene situation can be a cause for infections and other illnesses. Maintaining hygiene in the wild is one of the most difficult tasks. However, it has been made easier with the genius new products like alcohol hand sanitizers that have been proven to be very effective.

A final note on this section would be that you should always be aware of the inventory of the medical kit. It is essential that explorers check the kit before leaving each trip since each and every part of the kit is important to survival! In case any product is missing, then maintain hygiene and self-healing in the wild could become more uncomfortable.

Other Essentials

The most important essential for a wilderness trip would be the type of footwear and clothing items that explorers bring along. These depend on the type of weather that the forecast has revealed. Depending on the type of weather, different types of clothes can be packed. Always remember to pack more clothes than initially required to compensate for any emergencies, unplanned activities, or for having to spend extra days in the wild.

Clothing

One item that should be a permanent fixture in the exploration apparel is the footwear. A pair of hiking boots is perfect for all conditions and are also perfect for fending off spider and snake bites, as discussed in the chapter on wildlife. These boots provide adequate support on rocky trails and rugged terrain. In order to protect your feet from giving in after the trip, it is better to invest in a good pair of hiking shoes.

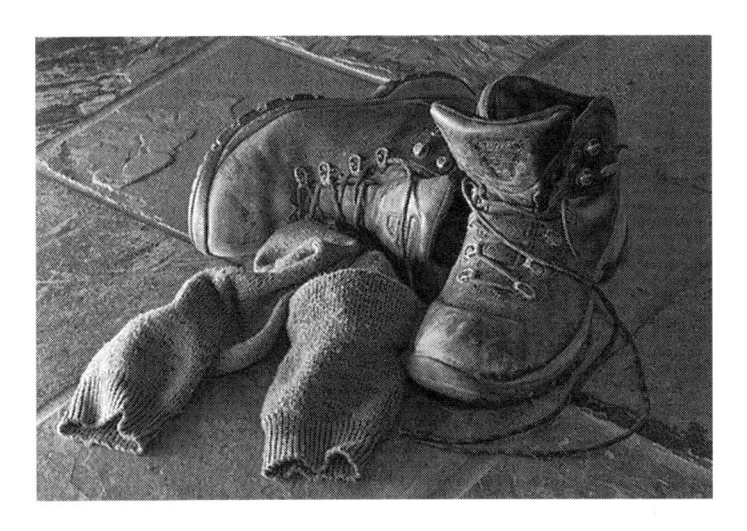

A lightweight jacket should also be kept in order to protect the upper body from the unforgiving winds that go around in the night. To protect the chest area from any infection, or even a cold, a jacket should be packed.

Additionally, to be stay protected from any rainy weather, the explorer should pack a sufficient amount of rainwear. This may include fleece pants, raincoats, warm jackets, and hats. Some gloves should also be packed to cover all parts of the body.

An essential part of the wilderness experience is to use nature for survival, and one such activity would be to find drinking water from the place that the explorer is visiting. It is essential that the explorer packs some kind of water purification system that will allow water from a water source to be made safe for drinking. Experts suggest that explorers should drink around half a liter of water for every hour that they are conducting their exploration activities. A backpacking stove, some dishes, and utensils must also be carried to sort out any cooking requirements.

For the primary shelter, a tent must be carried. This must be a full-fledged tent that can be manufactured by any company; however, it should fit the explorer's needs. A sleeping bag must also be kept with the tent as the added comfort is going to help ease the transition. The sleeping bag will also protect against the bugs that crawl over the ground.

Navigation Tools

The most important exploration tools are a map and a compass. These navigation tools are essential so that a new explorer does not get lost in a particular area. Along with these tools, it is necessary that a bushcraft knife has been kept in the back. The knife will be used in almost everything that an explorer does in the wild since it has such flexibility. It is also recommended that a pocket knife must also be kept to open cans and peel fruit and help in opening up small packages that are kept in the backpack.

As explained in the altitude sickness chapter, if an explorer wants to carry an inflatable oxygen tank, then he/she can pack that too.

However, that tool is only used for trekking and climbs to higher places. Such tools are also used by professionals who know how to use them as efficiently as possible. If this is your first time in the wilderness, then it is advisable that you follow the guidelines in each of the chapters rather than following other professionals.

The final thing to pack is this guide itself! This is the most comprehensive guide ever made on bushcraft. The wilderness aspect of nature is something that many people are afraid of, and through this guide, individuals are to be encouraged to become new explorers. By becoming explorers, you, too, can take part and witness the magical powers of nature. These powers are surreal, and as explained above, they have an important part to play in all of our lives.

These are the top essentials required to carry out an effective and fulfilling wilderness trip. If the backpack has some space, then a few personal items can be kept too! These items can vary from books to other things that help ease the explorer's mind it times of stress since the wild can sometimes become too much for even the experts to handle!

Conclusion

This book covers the most technical aspects of self-healing in the wilderness in the simplest way possible. The book is structured in a unique way, where the first few chapters tackle the wildlife of a certain area. Since the world is a very diverse place, not all regions could be covered in those chapters. However, most of the very common predators have been marked out for explorers so that they know how to self-heal if they come out of the wrong side in an encounter with these animals. The procedures are very easy to follow and require simple things to complete. The last chapter even has a complete list of items that are required to treat all kinds of bruises/wounds/fractures in the wild.

The wildlife also covers the types of plants and greenery that an explorer is going to encounter. An entire guide has been created to help explorers tackle the various ecosystems that they are going to face in their future trips. The self-healing procedures in this chapter are also easy to follow and have been simplified so that they are easier to perform. This is a one of a kind book that delivers on everything as it is a cross between a guide and a research study.

This resource also provides a new perspective on the phenomenon that is "bushcraft." That new perspective is the emotional and spiritual self-healing perspective. This new topic has been well researched upon for a couple of years now, and the details in that chapter open a new world for the majority of explorers that only focused on the physical part of bushcraft. However, the emotional aspect of this activity has a huge impact on the mental state of an individual. How can an individual explore these opportunities? Well, these questions have also been explored in order to give the entire picture of this activity.

The final chapter is a complete planning guide to a wilderness exploration trip. All sorts of logistical questions have been answered in that chapter in order to assure new explorers about their decisions. It is designed to encourage new explorers to pack efficiently and explore the wilderness at their own will. Not with anyone, but on their own!

New explorers that are afraid of the idea of going out into the wilderness alone can now address that issue head-on. All you need is this resource guide to go along in your backpack. If you follow all the important procedures and focus on all the important details given in this guide, then you have nothing to worry about!

Bibliography

Black, R. (2011, 08, 23). Species count put at 8.7 million. Retrieved 08 01, 2020, from https://www.bbc.com/news/: https://www.bbc.com/news/science-environment-14616161

Daniel, B. (2018, 06, 04). Spending time alone in nature is good for your mental and emotional health. Retrieved from https://theconversation.com: https://theconversation.com/spending-time-alone-in-nature-is-good-for-your-mental-and-emotional-health-92652

NHS. (2019, 07 08). Treatment Insect bites and stings. Retrieved from https://www.nhs.uk: https://www.nhs.uk/conditions/insect-bites-and-stings/treatment/

Universal Class. (2020). How to Treat Insect Bites and Illnesses in the Wilderness. Retrieved from https://www.universalclass.com: https://www.universalclass.com/articles/self-help/how-to-treat-insect-bites-and-illnesses-in-the-wilderness.htm

Williams, F. (2020). This is Your Brain on Nature. Retrieved 08 07, 2020, from https://www.nationalgeographic.com: https://www.nationalgeographic.com/magazine/2016/01/call-to-wild/

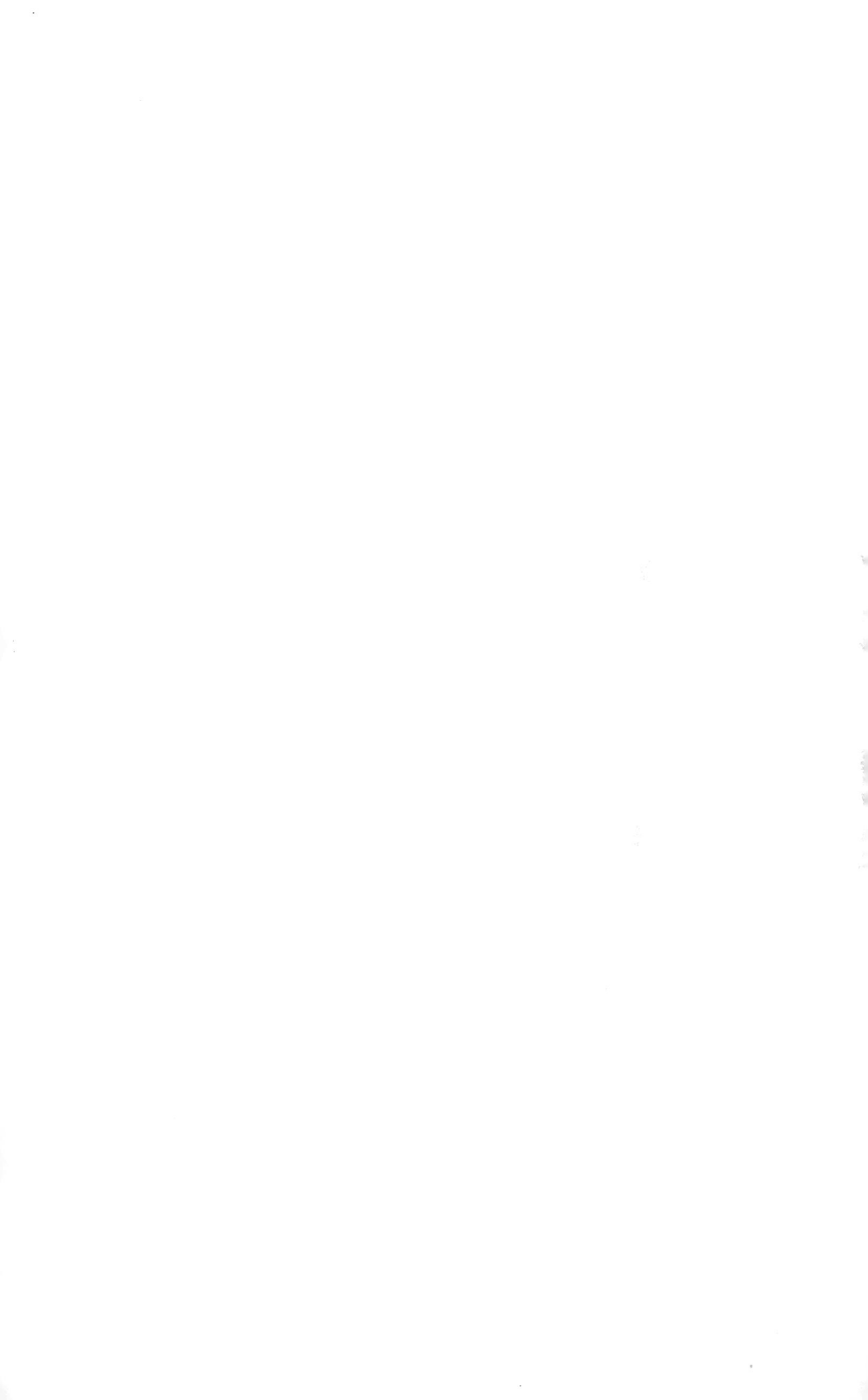

Printed in Great Britain
by Amazon